Miracle
Sugars

Miracle Sugars

The Glyconutrient Link to Disease Prevention and Improved Health

RITA ELKINS, M.H.

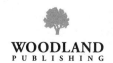

WOODLAND
PUBLISHING

The CIP data for this book is available from the Library of Congress.

For ordering information, contact:
Woodland Publishing, 448 East 800 North, Orem, Utah 84097
www.woodlandpublishing.com

ISBN 1-58054-367-7
Printed in the United States of America

The information in this book is for educational purposes only and is not recommended as a means of diagnosing or treating an illness. All matters concerning physical and mental health should be supervised by a health practitioner knowledgeable in treating that particular condition. Neither the publisher nor author directly or indirectly dispenses medical advice, nor do they prescribe any remedies or assume any responsibility for those who choose to treat themselves.

Contents

Introduction

I've been researching natural medicines for a long time. Over the years, I've compiled a short list of compounds I consider important enough to take myself. Recently, I added a group of nutrients, commonly called glyconutrients (and which I like to call the miracle sugars) to that preferential list. The word *glyconutrient* is a broad term used to describe many different kinds of beneficial plant sugars. The beneficial effects of glyconutrients on the human immune system are nothing less than remarkable. These glyconutrients profoundly impact the way our bodies defend against disease on a cell-to-cell basis. So much so, that their existence has prompted the development of a new science called glycobiology.

Unfortunately, few people know glyconutrients can make the difference between optimal or mediocre immune function. Why? Two reasons. First, anything called "sugar" has a well-deserved negative connotation. No one can deny that our societal obsession with sucrose (white sugar) has contributed to many serious health problems, ranging from obesity to diabetes.

Because I consider refined white sugar to be public health enemy number one, my first reaction to using supplemental "sugars" therapeutically to prevent and cure disease was, "you've go to be kidding." After doing my homework, I came to understand what ancient herbalists have known for generations—that plants rich in these special sugars fight disease.

Secondly, scientists have traditionally relegated the sugar or carbohydrate portion of a compound to the role of a mere "energy source." Virtually undetected and certainly underestimated until recently, glyconutrients offer us a new universe of possibilities in our quest to fight disease. Hundreds of studies link a deficiency of any one of these extraordinary sugars to everything from lupus to heart disease, ADHD, cancer and even infertility. Many more illnesses have been linked to an imbalance of these sugar molecules or the inability to utilize them properly. From mannose to beta-glucans, nature provides a marvelous array of sugars that, when ingested, work to construct superior disease resistance.

The average American diet supplies the body with only two sugars to any substantial degree (glucose and galactose), creating a new and unheard-of nutrient deficiency. The role of saccharides (another name for plant sugars) explains why specific plants were harvested and heralded as powerful cures for infection for millennia.

Naturally, the million-dollar question is whether the merits of these sugars justify their supplementation. A growing consensus among health experts suggests the answer is an emphatic "yes." A substantial body of evidence supports the notion that providing our immune network with certain sugars helps correct the chemical imbalances responsible for a harmful trend that is quickly becoming a global epidemic—dysfunctional immunity—the cause of a myriad of devastating diseases and syndromes. Moreover, it appears that correcting saccharide or sugar deficiencies may even help to reverse genetic code malfunctions that predispose a person to certain diseases.

Summary of What Glyconutrients Can Do

- decrease allergy symptoms
- lower cholesterol
- decrease body fat
- increase lean muscle mass
- enhance wound healing
- modulate autoimmune diseases (arthritis, lupus, psoriasis, type I diabetes, etc.)
- fight bacterial and viral infections
- ease symptoms of chronic fatigue syndrome/fibromyalgia
- lessen the toxic effects of radiation and chemotherapy
- augment the cancer-killing effect of conventional cancer treatments
- decrease depression
- help control some types of obesity

Personally, I believe that along with our daily vitamin, mineral and antioxidant array we should also take our daily dose of glyconutrients, which act as the essential building blocks of immunity. And so, I have chosen those sugars (compliments of Mother Nature) that I believe offer the most potential for optimal immune cell survival and function.

After years of researching complementary medicines, I've come to the conclusion that the cause of virtually every disease boils down to three things:

1. A malfunctioning immune system
2. Free radical damage from bad fats, bad chemicals, ultraviolet rays, and other toxins
3. The deficiency of one or more vital nutrients

Glyconutrients have the unique ability to address all three of these major modern-day health threats. At least eight simple glyconutrients (monosaccharides) are missing from most of our diets. The human body needs monosaccharides to function properly. These vital sugars combine with proteins and fats to create glycomolecules or glycoforms that coat the surface of virtually all cells. This "sugar coating" enables cell membranes to transfer messages to other cells. If we are missing any one of several crucial sugars, glycoprotein structures that help our immune system to function normally may be weakened or changed altogether. As a result, cellular messages may be full of errors.

Simply stated, the marriage of certain sugars with proteins and fats impacts virtually every biological function and may well be the single most important determiner of disease resistance. These plant sugars perform complex and sophisticated chemical actions, giving cells the ability to transfer coded messages that sustain life and maintain health.

The ultimate irony is that while most of us fail to consume enough of these desirable sugars, we are gorging ourselves on sugars that hurt our health. For me, understanding why aloe vera helps to heal, why echinacea fights infection and why medicinal mushrooms inhibit cancer all boils down to appreciating their glyconutrient content. Moreover, the ability of glucosamine to build cartilage, the immunoprotective action of breast milk and the reason ocean plants provide superior nutrition and disease protection also reflect the value of natural compounds rich in glyconutrients. Anyone who wants to build superior immunity needs to become acquainted with these sugars. The best place to start is with Chapter One.

The Family of Sugars: From Feast to Famine

"Just when you're beginning to think pretty well of people, you run across somebody who puts sugar on sliced tomatoes." –Will Cuppy

Imagine holding a sugar canister and feeding yourself thirty-five spoonsful of white sugar at one sitting. That's the amount a typical American consumes each and every day, and it's not all that hard to do. For example, a 12-ounce soda contains around 9 teaspoons of sugar alone and all of us are aware of our societal obsession with soft drinks. At this writing, the per-capita consumption of sugar in this country averages 130 pounds of sugar per person per year—a statistic that gives an entirely new meaning to the term *sweet tooth*. To make matters worse, hundreds of packaged foods contain hidden sugars that you may not even taste!

For example, sugar is routinely added to soups, peanut butter, macaroni and cheese, ketchup, mustard, bread and salad dressings, just to mention a few. And here's another sobering thought—some children consume more than 50 percent of their daily caloric intake as sugar. To illustrate—children start drinking soda pop at a deplorably young age (one to two years old). Toddlers drink an average of almost one cup of soda per day. And sugary cold cereals that kids continually snack on and eat for breakfast, lunch and dinner are also loaded with white sugar. The incidence of type II diabetes (once seen only in overweight, middle-aged people) is skyrocketing in American children. Because so many of our kids eat over half their caloric intake in the form of sugar, the World Health Organization (in response to rising rates of diabetes and obesity) has issued this guideline—people should consume no more than 10 percent of their calories from white sugar, also known as sucrose.

The Family of Sugar Molecules

When you digest that thirty-five spoonsful of sucrose each day, your body breaks it down into a simple sugar called glucose. Chemically speaking, glucose is a simple sugar—in other words, a monosaccharide. A monosaccharide cannot be reduced into a simpler molecule. Glucose (from plants and white sugar) and galactose (from milk) are the most common essential monosaccharides that we consume.

Monosaccharides are the basic building blocks of all sugars. Two monosaccharides join to form a disaccharide. Three to six monosaccharides join to form an oligosaccharide. Join a lot of monosaccharides (hundreds of thousands) and you have a polysaccharide. I can tell you that for most people, white sugar is the only sugar. The truth is that nature has engineered many different kinds of sugars. A sugar can range from a simple molecule to one that is much more complex. The number of hexose units a sugar contains determines its complexity. A hexose unit is the basic monosaccharide molecule containing six carbon atoms. For example, sucrose is a disaccharide, meaning it contains two hexose units.

The White Stuff

Those granular white crystals that sweeten up your menu are actually granules of bleached sucrose. Sucrose belongs to a general family of disaccharide sugars that include glucose, fructose, galactose, lactose, ribose and maltose. Sucrose is comprised of two monosaccharides, namely glucose and fructose. Fructose readily converts to glucose during the digestive process, so the end result of eating sucrose is glucose—a pure energy source for cells. While sucrose exists in nature, its bleached and altered form does not. Refined from cane or beet juice, all of the natural vitamins, minerals and fiber found in raw sugar are stripped away, leaving behind a sweet, high-calorie, virtually worthless food.

What Are Carbohydrates?

Carbohydrates are grouped into two categories: simple carbohydrates (sugars) and complex carbohydrates (starches). Simple carbohydrates, which convert to glucose quickly, can be found in milk, fruits and fruit juices, etc., while complex carbohydrates can be found in beans, pasta, grains and starchy vegetables like potatoes. Although carbohydrates may provide nutrients and fiber, all carbohydrates are eventually converted into glucose, which enters the blood as sugar and triggers insulin secretion from the pancreas. Granted, complex carbohydrates take longer to convert to glucose, but the fact remains—if you consume more carbohydrate calories than you can use, that sugar will be stored as glycogen or as fat. Each gram of carbohydrates is worth approximately four calories.

Because we typically overeat carbohydrates in the form of chips, cookies, cakes, pastries, soda, candy, sweetened cereals, etc., we add enormous amounts of empty calories to our metabolic furnace, which becomes over fueled resulting in the creation of fat. According to current statistics, carbohydrates make up from 500 to 700 of our consumed calories per day. Of equal importance, many of us obtain well over 1,000 calories from sweet or starchy foods daily. And seemingly nutritious foods like muffins and bagels can be chock full of sugar. In fact, someone once said a bagel is nothing more than an unsweetened doughnut with rigor mortis.

So what's the harm in a diet rich in carbs? Take a look at the biological journey a carbohydrate takes. It all starts with your first bite of that Twinkie.

1. A starchy or sugary food is consumed.
2. The food is chemically broken down into glucose.
3. Glucose enters the bloodstream. (Some is stored in the liver as glycogen for later use.)
4. Blood sugar rises.
5. The pancreas releases insulin, signaling body cells to take up and store excess glucose.
6. Blood sugar enters tissues on a cellular level.
7. Glucose is burned as fuel.
8. Blood sugar supply becomes exhausted.
9. Insulin levels drop.
10. Sugar reserves in the liver (glycogen) are released into the bloodstream as glucose.

Under normal circumstances, blood sugar remains fairly stable and glucose is used for immediate and stored energy. However, excessive carbohydrate intake can overwork the pancreas, causing problems. Blood sugar disorders like diabetes (high blood sugar) or hypoglycemia (low blood sugar) have been attributed to heavy carbohydrate loading on the pancreas. For instance, type II diabetics develop a resistance to the effects of insulin—a phenomenon some experts attribute to years of overeating carbohydrates. In this case, the pancreas produces insulin, but the body's cells are unable to use it; so it stays in the blood increasing the risk of obesity and heart disease. Individuals with hypoglycemia, on the other hand, may experience an excessive insulin response to carbohydrates that drives their blood sugar well below normal.

The Dark Side of White Sugar

Eating too much white sugar contributes to diabetes, insulin resistance, dental cavities, obesity and heart disease. In addition, a strong link exists among white sugar and ADHD and immune dysfunction. Furthermore, high blood sugar levels may boost free radical production, which can cause tissue damage and degenerative disease—explaining why diabetics have an increased risk of heart disease and circulatory problems. To illustrate—according to a study published in the *Journal of Clinical Endocrinology and Metabolism*, a drink containing 75 grams of pure glucose significantly increased the formation of free radicals in test subjects. Free radicals are biological bandits that steal molecules to stabilize themselves and in so doing, cause tissue damage and disease.

To make matters worse, eating sugar can deplete your body of B vitamins and minerals. Moreover, it can predispose people to energy and mood swings. I can tell you from personal experience that sugar sends me on an emotional roller coaster complete with energy highs and lows. Sugar also impairs digestion, stimulates hypoglycemic episodes and rots teeth. Unfortunately, curbing intense cravings for sugar can take some doing. Realizing that white sugar makes you feel lousy is a good place to start.

Can White Sugar Make You Sick?

When white sugar is consumed, phagocytes (the cells that eat bad guys for lunch) become less effective, thereby lowering our resistance to disease. Simply stated, eating white sugar weakens immune defenses—a fact that may explain why American children have such a high rate of ear infections, colds, etc. One study found that after eating white sugar, the efficacy of the immune system drops by 50 percent for up to forty-eight hours.

Significant amounts of B vitamins are actually required to metabolize and detoxify ingested sugar. Moreover, when you overload your body with sugar, you can inhibit the assimilation of nutrients from other foods. In other words, our bodies were not designed to cope with the enormous amounts of sugar we routinely consume. Consequently, too much sugar can generate a type of malnutrition that not only negatively impacts the body, but the mind as well. In addition, too much sugar can predispose us to yeast infections, aggravate some types of arthritis and asthma, cause tooth decay, elevate blood fats, and make us obese and diabetic.

Leo Galland, a physician and author of *Superimmunity for Kids*, says that the key to a strong, healthy immune system is optimal nutrition. If you want optimal protection from all kinds of infection, you have to cut down on sugar. Some mothers believe the sugar/immune link explains why their kids get sick after holidays like Halloween when their sugar consumption goes off the scale. So offer your kids cut up veggies, fruits and nuts instead of candy, chips and soda pop.

Is White Sugar Addictive?

Some experts believe that white sugar is addictive. In his book, *Sugar Blues*, William Dufty writes that the difference between sugar addiction and narcotic addiction is largely one of degree. Just ask anyone who tries to give up sugar cold turkey—they often experience fatigue, depression, moodiness, headaches, dizziness, muscle aches, etc. (all symptoms of drug withdrawal). Moreover, most people will tell you that the more sugar they eat, the more they crave. Equally important is the way sugar consumption and withdrawal affects behavior and mood. So is white sugar a drug? Perhaps it would be more accurate to refer to sugar as a substance that has a drug-like effect on the body. In and of itself, a moderate amount of sugar consumed now and then may be perfectly harmless. The potential problem, however, with eating a little sugar is that it stimulates our appetite for more sugar. Keep in mind also that if you abruptly cut off your sweet supply, you can feel depressed and edgy.

Tryptophan and phenylalanine (two important amino acids) compete with sugar for absorption in the intestines. These amino acids are the building blocks for brain chemicals that sustain mood. For this reason, nutritionists have long advised against eating protein and sugar at the same time because protein supplies our bodies with amino acids. Apparently, some people are more sensitive to sugar consumption as it relates to behavior and emotional state. Again, many mothers insist that their children become "wired" after eating too much sugar, although science has yet to document this effect.

The Glucose Glut

Although we typically overindulge in white sugar (our primary source of glucose), we fail to consume other essential sugars. Most people are completely unaware that other sugars exist in nature that support immune defenses. Granted, glucose provides energy for cellular functions, but that's about all. Ideally, we should be consuming an array of sugars provided by nature to enjoy maximum rather than minimum health. In fact, our failure to consume these nutrients is thought to be a major contributing factor to the dramatic increase seen in autoimmune disease and cancer over the last fifty years. The bottom line—feasting on sucrose (white sugar) starves our immune system, while providing it with essential saccharides fortifies it.

In addition to consuming sucrose, most Americans also consume excessive amounts of fructose (fruit sugar) and galactose (milk sugar). These single simple sugars require little or no digestion and are easily absorbed directly into the bloodstream—an action that can prompt excessive insulin secretion, which may contribute to unstable blood sugar levels. The link between these sugars and heart disease, obesity, and behavioral disorders is disturbing. A growing body of evidence shows that excessive consumption of these sugars is connected to the rise of several degenerative diseases typically seen in Western cultures.

A Note on Artificial Sweeteners

Okay. You have a sweet tooth that won't be denied—so is the solution to switch to an artificial sweetener? Not necessarily. Having received the FDA stamp of approval, compounds like aspartame and saccharin are routinely consumed with little thought given to their health risks. Andrew Weil, M.D., writes in his book, *Natural Health Natural Medicine:*

"More worrisome than preservatives are artificial sweeteners. Saccharin, a known carcinogen, should be avoided. Cyclamates, banned some years ago for suspected carcinogenicity, are not being reconsidered for use in food. They taste better than saccharin but cause diarrhea in some people. Recently, aspartame

(NutraSweet) has become enormously popular. The manufacturer portrays it as a gift from nature, but, although the two component amino acids occur in nature, aspartame itself does not. Like all artificial sweeteners, aspartame has a peculiar taste. Because I have seen a number of people, mostly women, who report headaches from this substance, I don't regard it as being free from toxicity. Women also find that aspartame aggravates PMS (premenstrual syndrome). I think you are better off using moderate amounts of sugar than consuming any artificial sweeteners on a regular basis."

While thousands of Americans continue to consume aspartame in unprecedented amounts, controversy surrounding its safety lingers. Dr. Richard Wurtman of the Massachusetts Institute of Technology (MIT) has reported that abnormal concentrations of neurotransmitters developed when he fed laboratory animals large doses of aspartame. He believes that the phenylalanine content of the sweetener actually manipulates and alters certain brain chemicals, which could initiate behavioral changes and even seizures. He also suggests that while small quantities of aspartame may be safe, the cumulative effects of the compound, particularly if consumed with high-carbohydrate, low-protein snacks, could be serious.

Aspartame has been marketed as a safe substance for the general public—except for those few individuals who suffer from PKU (phenylketonuria), a relatively rare disorder. Most consumers assume that aspartame is a perfectly benign compound and use it liberally. It is, in fact, comprised of phenylalanine, aspartic acid and methanol (wood alcohol). As previously mentioned, the various side effects associated with the ingestion of aspartame include migraines, memory loss, slurred speech, dizziness, stomach pain and even seizures.

In addition, because aspartame contains chemicals that affect brain cell function, significant questions have been raised concerning its link to increased incidence of brain tumors. Acesulfame K, another artificial sweetener on the market, has also been linked to cancer by the Center for Science in the Public Interest. In spite of these findings, these sweeteners have been approved by the FDA and are recognized as safe.

Using Stevia as a Sugar Substitute

Stevia may well be the safest of the non-caloric sweeteners. As a natural herbal sweetener, stevia has all the benefits of artificial sweeteners and none of the drawbacks. It can be added to a variety of foods to make them sweet without adding calories or impacting the pancreas or adrenal glands. It can also satisfy carbohydrate cravings without interfering with blood sugar levels or adding extra pounds. Using stevia to create treats for children is also another excellent way to avoid weight gain, tooth decay and possible hyperactivity. While it may take some getting used to initially, stevia products are becoming easier to measure and better tasting.

When the whole leaf extract or powdered forms of stevia make contact with the tongue, the resulting taste can be described as a sweet, slightly licorice-like and transient bitter flavor. If stevia is used correctly with hot water or other liquid, both of these flavors will disappear. At this writing, researchers are working on a new extraction process that will preserve stevia's sweetening potency while minimizing any aftertaste associated with the herb.

Chapter Two

Glyconutrients:
Beneficial Sugars

"If you don't do what's best for your body, you're the one who
comes up on the short end." *-Julius Erving*

Collectively, sugars that benefit human health are often referred to as glyconutrients. *Glyco* refers to sweet. Hence, a glyconutrient is a biochemical that contains a sugar molecule. The prefix *glyco* can be placed in front of a fat or protein and suggests that a sugar is attached to the molecule. Chemists now believe that at least eight dietary sugars (also called saccharides or carbohydrates) play a profound role in the maintenance of human health. These sugars are emerging as critical carbohydrate compounds. When these sugars pair up with proteins, they form glycoproteins (compounds that keep the immune communications system sharp). Unlike white sugar, these plant sugars contribute to cellullar protection from microbial invaders and autoimmune syndromes rather than encouraging a less healthy state.

The study of glyconutrient-containing molecules as they pertain to human health is still in its infancy, and yet its implications are stunning. To date, a great deal of scientific evidence suggests that consuming certain obscure plant sugars found in nature work to direct the action of immune cells. Over the last decade, research has revealed sugars that coat cell surfaces (glycoforms) enable cells to talk to each other. The word *glycoform* is a broad term for large molecules that are made when sugars combine with proteins or fats. When sugars combine with a fat molecule, a glycolipid is formed. When sugars combine with a protein molecule, a glycoprotein is formed.

Glycoproteins and glycolipids cover the surface of every cell in your body and serve as telephone lines between cells. Make no mistake. There is no way to overestimate what glycoproteins and glycolipids do for you. The proper relay of information between cells determines your health status. Your immune cells cannot relay vital messages without these glycoforms, and your body cannot create enough glycoforms without sufficient levels of the essential eight glyconutrients, which are glucose, mannose, galactose, xylose, fucose, N-acetylglucosamine, N-acetylgalactosamine and N-acetylneuraminic acid.

Because we no longer eat a wide array of plants, nuts, seeds and other whole foods, it's not hard to believe many of us lack specific glyconutrients that support immunity. Glyconutrient supplementation is a great way to bridge the gap between the ideal diet and the realistic diet.

Again, we cannot underestimate the importance of getting sufficient levels of these potentially life-saving nutrients. The essential eight sugars are engineered to instruct your immune cells where to go and what to kill. They play an important role in preventing a number of disorders—from allergies to asthma and from cancer to chronic fatigue.

Cells, both good and bad, often sport a carbohydrate cover. In other words, both proteins and fats can contain a sugar molecule as part of their chemical structure. And so can microbial invaders. This sugar "coating" of glycoforms enables an immune defense cell to bind with microbial invaders and antibodies. You can imagine the profound role that this "binding" plays in the process of fighting off invaders. Substantial data suggests that when cells "hook up" they do so with their sugar-coated portions. Infectious agents bind to healthy cells in the same way. Quite simply that's how we get sick—glycoforms on microbes and viruses bind to our healthy cells. The notion behind therapeutic saccharide supplementation is simple. When we eat foods containing the essential eight sugars, those sugar molecules help the immune system block the sugar receptors of more undesirable organisms such as bacteria or viruses, thereby decreasing the extent or duration of an infection, without any of the potentially dangerous side effects of a drug.

Glycobiology: Cutting-Edge Science

Glycobiology refers to a relatively new field of study that looks at saccharide compounds and how they impact health. Research into glyconutrients reveals a multifaceted subject that studies the diverse effects of sugars on cellular functions and disease. "Sugars in particular perform an astonishing range of jobs. Once regarded mainly as energy-yielding molecules (glucose and glycogen) and as structural elements, they are now known to combine with proteins and fats on cell surfaces and, so situated, influence cell-to-cell communications, the functioning of the immune system, the ability of various infectious agents to make us sick and the progression of cancer," says Thomas Maeder, a well-known glyconutrients researcher, in a recent issue of *Scientific American.*

Glycobiologists are currently investigating the sugar portion of proteins and fats. They have discovered that sugar-bound proteins work to keep our hormones in balance, fight off disease invaders, enable blood to clot, give our cells their structural support network and, perhaps most important of all, create a complex cellular messaging system.

Like so many new frontiers in science, the role of these sugars will expand in the future. Unfortunately, until recently, these sugars got no respect from the scientific community and were often thought of as nothing more than contaminants, or at best, simple energy sources. To be fair, one reason so many scientists failed to explore the world of glycobiology is that sugars come in a vast array of chemical "clothing," making it extremely difficult to decipher their chemical codes. Consequently, the task was relegated to the back burner. Today, with the availability of new technology, scientists are able to delve into the world of glyconutrients, and they are discovering what ancient medical practitioners already knew—that specific plant sugars exert extraordinary actions on the human immune system. Glyconutrients enable cells to transmit vital data to other cells. When it comes to the immune system, clear and uncorrupted communication is vital when disease-causing organisms enter the body.

Hundreds of monosaccharides (simple sugars) are found in various plants. While monosaccharides are discussed in this book, so are polysaccharides (complex sugars). In fact, I have attempted to cover all the saccharides or sugars I believe offer remarkable immune-boosting properties.

Sweets That Aren't Sweet

Be aware that just because something is called a "sugar" doesn't mean it has a sweet taste. In fact many sugars have no taste at all or if they do, they are usually a bit on the bitter side. In addition, unlike sucrose, glyconutrients don't raise insulin levels or add pounds. In fact, there is some evidence that they may even prompt weight loss. Glyconutrients fill several other very important roles in the body. In addition to regulating blood sugar levels, they

- work against tumors
- boost immune activity and efficiency
- heal damaged tissue
- complement chemotherapy and radiation
- ease joint inflammation
- repair cartilage
- boost brain function
- lower bad cholesterol
- increase bone density
- ease hormone-driven disorders (PMS and menopause)
- repair mucosal linings
- regulate overactive immune responses (autoimmune disease)

A New Generation of Glycodrugs?

Because health experts are now recognizing the tremendous potential of these sugars, in October of 2001, the National Institutes of Health awarded a five-year, multi-million dollar grant to the Consortium for Functional Glyconomics, (investors dedicated to developing synthetic sugar chains for use in pharmaceutical drugs). The term *glycomics* is a new word that refers to the study of sugars produced in an organism or cell. Experts realize that utilizing these sugars in drugs could work to regulate hormones, direct cellular traffic and regulate the immune system. Many scientists believe that the answers to disease prevention lies in the field of glycomics, which could spawn the creation of a new class of important drugs. While past sugar-based drugs don't have a stellar track record, a new emphasis on their potential has revitalized researchers. Inevitably, due to recent technology, a new generation of "sugar-laced" medications will certainly result. Current breakthroughs in the ability to decode these sugars have opened the door to innovative ways to synthesize and use "glycoside" medicines.

Obviously, the therapeutic potential of glycodrugs is enormous. They could include future cancer vaccinations and potent infection and inflammation fighters. In addition, sugar-based drugs may be able to treat autoimmune diseases and a number of mysterious disorders. Keep in mind that many prescription drugs are already considered "glycosides." Ironically, in the rush to develop glycodrugs, dietary supplement companies have beaten the pharmaceutical industry to the punch. Having recognized the tremendous potential of these sugars, experts in the natural health field have already designed glyconutrient supplements that are readily available to the consumer now.

Have You Had Your Sugars Today?

It's common knowledge that supplementing the body with vitamin A, vitamin C, and zinc can boost immunity. Now the emergence of immune-boosting substances like transfer factors from colostrum, polysaccharide-rich herbs and isolated glyconutrients forces us to rethink how we can maximize immune defenses. Scores of studies substantiate the crucial role that these natural compounds play in tailoring our immune responses to microbial invaders. Concerning immune function, glyconutrients do three things.

First, they boost our resistance to disease by giving microbes and viruses fewer places to set up shop. Second, they fortify our ability to fight disease by boosting the ability of our immune cells to find and fight foreign agents. And third, they decrease our recovery time by increasing the body's ability to heal itself.

The notion of taking these sugars in supplement form as part of an overall dietary protocol may have real value when it comes to disease prevention and recovery. Should these sugars be taken on a "one-a-day" basis? Read on.

Glyconutrients: The More, the Merrier

The higher your intake of glyconutrients, the more raw materials your body has to balance its immune cell networks. In other words, when you consume critical plant sugars, you give your body the best fighting chance to heal itself. Moreover, the presence of these sugars helps to stimulate the action of other biochemicals that sweep up dangerous free radicals. By so doing, damage to cells is minimized. The presence of disease or injury can generate more free radicals, which damage tissue and raise the risk of malignancy. No pharmaceutical drug can prompt these kinds of marvelous reactions—a fact that emphasizes that when given the right tools, the human body has an enormous capacity to correct itself. As mentioned earlier, ancient medical practitioners knew that certain plants prompted these reactions, although they didn't know why—we know why and yet have failed to take full advantage of glyconutrient compounds as legitimate medicinal agents.

Glyconutrient Sources

Certain plant parts, fruits, yeasts, molds and other fungi naturally contain glyconutrients. You'll recognize some of these sugar sources as quite well-known herbs, while others may be unfamiliar. Some common sources of glyconutrients include the following:

- aloe vera
- *Cordyceps sinensis*
- coriolus mushroom
- echinacea
- astragalus
- reishi and shiitake mushrooms

- yeasts
- saps
- woods
- husks
- breast milk
- pectins (gum acacia)
- shellfish
- bovine cartilage
- bovine colostrum
- maize

Note: Many of the above substances have long been recognized as botanical immune-system boosters.

The Essential Eight Sugars

Out of all the medicinal sugars found in nature, a growing body of evidence suggests that eight of them play the greatest role in maximizing the cellular messaging network of the immune system. Why? Because these are the specific sugars that combine with protein molecules to create glycoproteins (major cellular communicators) and other glyco-compounds.

The essential eight sugars are found on the surface of cells and are involved in the process of cellular recognition. They are crucial for the production of immune glycoproteins and proper cell function. The essential eight are also produced by plants that most of us don't consume today. While it's true that simple glucose and galactose (sugars we get plenty of) can be converted into some of these important sugars, the presence of disease, medications, pollutants or free radicals can impair the process. For this reason, some scientists speculate that the body fails to keep up with the demand to produce glycoproteins—a scenario that could compromise immune function.

In 1998, scientists at the University of California at Irvine determined that eight monosaccharides are required for the creation of glycoproteins. According to *Harper's Biochemistry Textbook*, the essential eight are the following:

- glucose
- galactose
- fucose
- mannose
- xylose
- N-acetylneuraminic acid
- N-acetylglucosamine
- N-acetylgalactosamine

Glucose is readily available in our diets (it's converted from white sugar, fructose and starchy foods) and in most cases is oversupplied in the form of sugar cane, rice, corn, potatoes, wheat and other starchy foods. Glucose enters the bloodstream rapidly, helps to fuel brain function, contributes to calcium absorption, enhances cellular communication and provides a quick source of energy. Ingesting too much glucose can cause obesity and type II diabetes. Insulin resistance and even arteriosclerosis have also been linked to high blood sugar or glucose levels. Deranged glucose metabolism has also been implicated in mental disorders and binge eating. While glucose is vital to survival, most of us have no trouble keeping our bodies well supplied. In fact, our overconsumption of sucrose and starchy, refined foods has resulted in dangerous blood sugar disorders.

Galactose is obtained from the conversion of lactose (milk sugar) and is also easily obtained from dairy products (unless you suffer from lactose intolerance). Galactose contributes to wound healing, inhibits inflammation and boosts calcium absorption. It also exerts significant antitumor activity.

Interestingly, a lack of galactose has been linked with some autoimmune diseases.

Fucose is readily found in breast milk and in several medicinal mushrooms. It has numerous well-documented benefits for the immune system including the normalization of overactive immune function. In addition, it also works to inhibit tumor growth and spreading. Fucose is also profoundly important for efficient neuron transmission in the brain. The inability to use or metabolize fucose properly has been connected to a number of diseases (cancer, diabetes, some viral infections, etc.).

Mannose plays a profound role in cellular interactions and can naturally lower blood sugar levels. Mannose is absolutely vital for proper immune defense against microbial invaders. It also has a natural anti-inflammatory effect. In addition, mannose contributes to tissue regeneration, inhibits tumor growth and fights bacterial, viral, parasitic, and fungal infections. Your ability to heal depends on the presence of mannose and if you have lupus, you'll be interested to know that a mannose deficiency has been linked to the disease.

Xylose is often included in sugarless gums and candies as xylitol because it has a sweet taste but does not cause tooth decay. Recently, xylose has been added to nasal sprays because it appears to discourage the binding of allergens and pathogens to mucous membranes. It also has known antibacterial and antifungal properties and may help prevent certain cancers. One more added bonus is that using it in gum and nasal sprays appears to discourage the incidence of ear infections in children.

N-acetylneuraminic acid is another sugar abundantly found in breast milk that dramatically impacts brain function and growth. It also boosts immune function and has documented antiviral and antibacterial actions making it a powerful pathogen fighter. In fact, this sugar has the documented ability to inhibit the replication of various flu viruses. It also appears to lower LDL cholesterol. Research shows that in certain disease states, the ability to digest this sugar is impaired.

N-acetylglucosamine is particularly beneficial for cartilage regeneration and joint inflammation. Glucosamine (a well-known natural medicine for arthritic conditions), is extracted from this sugar compound. The chemistry of this sugar prompts the production of cartilage, thereby improving joint mobility and discomfort. In addition, it also has significant antitumor activity and several other therapeutic effects. Deficiencies or malfunctions in the ability to metabolize this sugar have been linked to diseases of the bowel.

N-acetylgalactosamine is the least known of the eight sugars, although it appears to inhibit the growth of some tumors and, like the other sugars, plays an individual role in keeping cell communications clear and promptly delivered. Research on this particular sugar has been limited.

The Skinny on the Essential Eight

Concerning these special sugars, consider this quote made in 1998 and published in *Metabolism*, "Each of these eight sugars links up with specific proteins to activate different types of cascade or chain reactions. Interestingly, galactose and mannose convert directly into glycoproteins, without having to break down into glucose first. The conclusion—glyconutrients may provide a whole new class of cell nutrients that may be preferable to glucose." It is the availability of these sugars that prompts a variety of cellular reactions, including 1) the release of immune substances, 2) the phagocytosis of bacteria and cellular debris, 3) the inhibition of the spread of malignant cells, and 4) the prevention of bacterial and viral binding to the surface.

Where Are the Essential Eight Sugars Found?

Earlier in this chapter, I gave you a list of the most common sources of the essential eight sugars. You might have noticed that some of those sources aren't readily available. For example, not too many grocery stores sell tree sap these days. Still, there are some glyconutrient sources that are more common. They include the following:

- aloe vera
- breast milk
- bread molds
- mushrooms
- arabinogalactans
- pectins

Other Important Sugar Sources

Other sugars found in plants like medicinal mushrooms and blue-green algaes also offer a wide array of therapeutic benefits and include the following:

- acemannan
- beta-glucans
- chitins and chitosan
- lentinan
- maitake d-fraction
- inulin and oligofructose
- polysaccharide K and P

- ling zhi-8
- bovine tracheal cartilage

Xylitol

Xylitol is a white crystalline substance that for all purposes looks and tastes like white sugar. Unlike synthetic sugar substitutes, xylitol is not an artificial compound, therefore it is readily accepted by the human body. Xylitol exists in tiny amounts in fruits, berries and mushrooms. Because xylitol is slowly absorbed into the bloodstream and is only partially metabolized, it has a much lower caloric value—about 40 percent lower, in fact—than white sugar. For this reason, it can be used in certain amounts by diabetics.

Xylitol is commonly found in chewing gums and is considered a food additive. Its inclusion in chewing gum is especially beneficial since it appears to reduce tooth decay. Moreover, several studies show that xylitol can stop or even reverse dental caries, and this effect appears to be long term. Sugar-free chewing gums and candies that contain xylitol have already been endorsed by several dental associations. Of equal importance, xylitol nose sprays may also discourage ear infections in children. In this application, it works by inhibiting the growth of a bacteria called *Streptococcus pneumoniae*.

A study published in a 1996 issue of the *British Medical Journal*. The trial involved over 306 children with a history of ear infections. Half of the children chewed xylitol-containing gum at a rate of two pieces several times daily after meals and snacks. The other half chewed ordinary gum. Over a sixty-day period, 21 percent of the regular gum chewers as opposed to 12 percent of the xylitol group, came down with one or more ear infections. Interestingly, just chewing gum seems to prevent ear infections by clearing fluid from the ear canals; however, the presence of white sugar in the gum may also stimulate the growth of bacteria. The xylitol-chewing children experienced almost a 50 percent drop in ear infections because it not only kept fluid flowing in the ear canals, it inhibited the growth of infectious bacteria. Although xylitol is considered safe, it can cause diarrhea. If you're using it to sweeten foods in granular form, you may have to adjust your dosages until you adapt.

Sorbitol

Like xylitol, sorbitol is a natural sweetener (technically referred to as a polyol, or sugar alcohol) that has significantly less calories than sucrose or table sugar and does not promote tooth decay. Discovered by a French chemist in 1872, it occurs naturally in an assortment of fruits and berries. Today sorbitol is produced commercially and can be purchased in liquid or granular form. It is frequently found in a variety of food products and is considered very safe. It's not only used to sweeten foods, but it also adds an appealing texture and is approximately 60 percent as sweet as sucrose, with one-third fewer calories. Sorbitol is used by diabetics and, due to its humectant property, is often placed in skin-smoothing cosmetics. Interestingly, when added to charcoal, sorbitol is also able to block the absorption of certain ingested poisons. In women, sorbitol appears to mitigate the symptoms of PMS, although we don't understand how.

Mannitol

In chemical terms, mannitol is the alcohol form of the sugar mannose. It occurs naturally in pineapples, olives, asparagus, sweet potatoes and carrots and is extracted from seaweed for use as a food additive. It also has sweetening power; so like xylitol and sorbitol, it is also found in commercial food products suitable for diabetic consumption.

Studies also confirm its surprising ability to reduce damage to injured kidneys and boost blood flow after aneurysm surgery. It also has the ability when used therapeutically to cleanse the colon. Several other studies confirm the ability of

Why Don't Doctors Use Therapeutic Sugars?

All that most doctors know about sugars is that they are burned for energy. End of story. You won't find a chapter on glycobiology in a medical student's biochemistry textbook. One reason is because much of the health potential of these sugars has only recently emerged. Another reason is the hesitancy of the medical profession to acknowledge the therapeutic use of nutrients rather than bona-fide prescription drugs. Ironically, while scores of studies on the various actions of glyconutrients fill PubMed compilations, the majority of doctors have no idea what they do or how to use them.

mannitol to inhibit the *Heliobacter pylori* bacteria linked with the formation of gastric ulcers and others. It also has the ability to gather dangerous free radicals, which qualifies it as an antioxidant.

Ending the Famine

When cells are given a variety of sugars to work with, the speed and efficiency of their cellular contact is greatly enhanced. In other words, they become well directed. On the other hand, when we lack certain plant sugars, the immune system can be likened to a slow Internet connection that struggles to load web pages and fails to recognize important links. Consequently, sites may be skipped and data may be transferred at a painfully slow rate. Adding more RAM to the computer can correct the problem.

The same is true for our cellular "Web sites." When our sugar profile is incomplete, cells can become misguided, sluggish or even confused, as if to say "message does not compute." When this happens, we can become susceptible to disease. To make matters worse, our ability to heal can become dangerously compromised. Providing the body with a continual supply of glyconutrients helps avoid this cellular communication meltdown. Glyconutrients bind to proteins and embed themselves into cellular membranes, giving cells that may not understand each other a better bio-language.

Chapter Three

Don't Be a Good Host: The Great Immune Depression

"You can set yourself up to be sick, or you can
choose to stay well." *–Wayne Dyer*

Have you noticed all the new "syndromes" that have been added to current medical encyclopedias? Mysterious maladies continue to surface, and most of them have no known cause. From chronic fatigue syndrome to fibromyalgia to ADHD, it seems like a new disease or condition pops up every year. Many of these ailments consist of a bizarre cluster of symptoms that cannot be categorized. Sadly many of these diseases dramatically compromise the quality of life for thousands of people.

Moreover, allergies, ear infections and disorders like sinusitis are escalating, suggesting that our immune systems have either degraded or have become dangerously overactive. Personally, I have come to believe that many syndromes not currently linked to infectious organisms are, in reality, caused by an immune system that has gone awry.

Your immune defenses may be working well below capacity. In fact, we are learning that a malfunctioning immune system can be the real and silent cause of everything from heart disease to obesity. Many experts believe that immune system dysfunction is the greatest health threat we face. Research studies indicate that over the last few decades, our natural killer cell defenses have been weakened—a fact that may explain why we face an onslaught of mystery syndromes. Simply put, our immune systems have been overworked and underpaid.

The Immune System: Seek and Destroy

The immune system defends the body from attack by invaders that it designates as foreign. Characterized by an elaborate and ever-adapting communication network, the immune system continually patrols the body. Its mission statement can be summarized in three words—recognize, respond and remember. Immune cells must recognize and then react appropriately to structures called antigens. Antigens can be found on infectious organisms or on the body's own cells. Being able to tell the difference is crucial.

Warrior T and B Cells

The majority of cells found in the immune system are white blood cells and they consist of various types. T and B cells belong to a class called lymphocytes. T cells work to eradicate infected cells and communicate with other cells to sharpen the immune response to a threat. B cells produce antibodies, which stick to an antigen and actually flag it for destruction by other immune cells. Macrophages and neutrophils circulate throughout the body and act as sentinels continually watching for foreign invaders. In the event that one is discovered, these cells surround the cell or substance and destroy it by releasing toxic molecules. When immune dysfunction occurs, these toxic compounds can also damage healthy tissue—a phenomena seen in some types of autoimmune disease. Certain molecules inhabit the surface of all our cells and participate in the vast communication network that alerts other immune cells to come to the rescue. The germ-killing compounds secreted by T cells are called cytokines and chemokines. Cytokines are proteins that have the ability to command other immune cells to attack, multiply or die. Once again, if these cytokines become unregulated, autoimmune diseases can result. Chemokines refer to tiny cytokine molecules that act as a magnet for other immune cells, and they too can cause autoimmune disease if they go unchecked.

B cells clear away foreign antigens by binding to the antigen or by producing designer antibodies that seek and destroy specific antigens. B cells can only make antibodies after receiving the right signal from a T cell. When B cells get the wrong info and make antibodies against the antigens found on healthy tissues, autoimmune diseases can occur (for more detail, refer to chapter on autoimmune disease). While the incidence of autoimmune disease (an overactive immune system) seems to be on the rise, underactive or compromised immunity is also rampant.

Natural Killer Cells on the Decline

Another type of lymphocyte is the natural killer (NK) cell and they appear to be on the decline. Stated simply, our immune arsenals are getting low on ammunition. NK cells provide our first line of defense against invaders. A low NK cell count means a much higher risk of disease and tissue degeneration. Today we're actually able to measure natural killer cell counts, and the news isn't good. For a variety of reasons, many of our immune defenders are not up to snuff. Sadly, too many people with compromised immunity remain unaware that certain natural compounds coupled with good nutrition can improve immune function. Significant evidence shows that glyconutrient supplementation can substantially increase NK cell activity both in healthy people and in people with compromised immune systems. Taking a variety of key supplements combined with good nutrition and exercise gives a person an amazing advantage over someone who ignores the demands of the immune system, or worse yet, abuses that system.

Eating Ourselves to Death

Henry Miller said that Americans will eat garbage, provided you sprinkle it liberally with ketchup. Unfortunately, our "undiscriminating" palates have prompted us to fill up on foods full of empty calories. In fact, some experts believe that when it comes to nutrition and health, humans were better off during the "dark ages," when we ate little meat and lots of whole grains, fruits and vegetables that were in season. Today we load our stomachs with empty calories and synthetic chemicals that deprive us of essential vitamins, minerals, fiber and crucial plant nutrients. Consequently, we suffer from obesity, diabetes, heart disease and cancer. In an age when food is plentiful, the notion that people in this country might be mineral deficient is absurd. Even a mild deficiency of iron and selenium (both of which Americans are typically low in) can suppress immune function. Minerals are obtained from vegetables and fruits grown in mineral-rich soil. The fact that we fail to eat enough fruits and veggies, coupled with their growth in nutrient-poor soil, suggests that mineral deficiency is a real cause for concern.

Overindulging in fats poses another threat to the immune system. Most of us eat diets high in an assortment of bad fats. Interestingly, in a surprising 1993 report published in

Progressive Food and Nutrition, scientists found that excessive fat intake impairs immunity. Moreover, high-fat diets can contribute to obesity. The number of obese Americans continues to grow despite the availability of gyms and diet foods. Approximately 60 percent of adults are overweight or obese, as are almost 13 percent of children. Furthermore, the number of Americans with preventable diseases, such as type II diabetes and heart disease is on the rise.

Currently, about three hundred thousand people die each year from illnesses related to being overweight, and many of us suffer from nutrient deficiencies, even though we have year-round access to a wide variety of foods. The truth is, while we are gaining ground in some health arenas, we are losing ground in others.

Malnutrition Amid Plenty

Much of the food we consume today has been fragmented, chemically altered and unnaturally preserved. In addition, we're now eating nonfood substitutes as if they were the real thing. Most of us would agree that Americans eat way too much junk food and snack on sweet, fatty, calorie-laden foods. What we call food today sometimes stretches the imagination. Michael Jacobson, in the April 1975 edition of *Smithsonian* states:

"Benjamin Franklin and Abraham Lincoln, if they could visit us, would probably have some difficulty distinguishing between a toy store and a supermarket. They would not even recognize as foods such products as artificial whipped cream in its pressurized can, or some breakfast cereals that are almost half sugar and bear little resemblance to cereal grains."

Over the last thirty years, modern technology has changed what we eat and the way we eat it. We now routinely consume new crop varieties that have been genetically engineered, hormone-fattened beef and poultry, foods that have undergone a number of high-tech processing techniques, and a wide variety of food additives and preservatives.

Foods are no longer eaten in season as in past generations. Fruits and vegetables are shipped transcontinentally and are often packed in dry ice or refrigerated for extended periods of time. In addition, new foods have been created and synthetic food substitutes like artificial sweeteners and synthetic fats are rapidly dominating commercially packaged foods.

The immune impact of this kind of eating is impossible to assess but it is significant, to say the least. Even in the good old days of the fifties and sixties, a typical dinner consisted of a slab of red meat, boiled veggies, potatoes and gravy, white bread and margarine, red jello and pudding for dessert. The advent of canned foods and frozen TV dinners (by the way, Johnny Carson said if it weren't for Philo T. Farnsworth, the inventor of television, we'd still be eating frozen radio dinners) took the nation by storm and fresh foods took second place to "convenience" foods.

Many families on tight budgets ate plenty of filling leftovers like pot roast or creamed potatoes that were served over and over. I remember someone saying that the most remarkable thing about their mother is that for thirty years she served the family nothing but leftovers and the original meal has never been found. In any event, our eating habits have been going downhill for decades, and we need to rewind the tape. Unfortunately, our digestive systems have become accustomed to salty, fatty, overcooked, and processed foods. Our only hope for change is to retrain our palates to savor foods custom-made by Mother Nature. Study after study verifies that when we supply our bodies with the necessary dietary building blocks, we give ourselves a fighting chance against the assault and battery our bodies deal with every day.

Nutrition and the Immune System: From Birth to Old Age

A study recently published in the *European Journal of Clinical Nutrition* found that protein malnutrition is associated with a significant impairment of cell-mediated immunity, phagocyte function and antibody concentrations. In fact, the trial showed that a deficiency of various single nutrients results in altered immune response, even when the deficiency was relatively mild. Specifically, micronutrients such as zinc, selenium, iron, copper, vitamins A, C, E and B6, and folic acid profoundly impacted immune response. Interestingly, scientists also discovered that overeating and obesity also reduced immunity. Of equal importance, the study found that low-birth-weight infants have a prolonged impairment of cell-mediated immunity that can be partly restored by providing extra amounts of dietary zinc. In the elderly, impaired immunity can be enhanced by supplementing modest amounts of a combination of micronutrients.

It Just Ain't What It Used to Be

That gorgeous, green produce you're adding to your shopping cart probably isn't all it's cracked up to be. The notion that we are getting all the nutrients we need from eating plenty of fruits and veggies is rapidly losing ground. Mineral-depleted soils and nutritionally "dead" foods are scientifically valid issues that raise concern over the real nutrient content of produce. In an issue of *August Celebration*, Linda Grover made a very enlightening yet alarming statement. She said, "In 1948 you could buy spinach that had 158 milligrams of iron. But by 1965, the maximum iron they could find had dropped to 27 milligrams. In 1973, it was averaging 2.2. milligrams. That's down from 150. That means today you'd have to eat seventy-five bowls of spinach to get the same amount of iron that one bowl might have given you back in 1948. That explains why Popeye was so big and so strong, right?" I don't know about you, but I was stunned by that piece of information. What it told me was that mineral supplementation is absolutely essential today. And it's important to know that a deficiency of even just one vitamin or mineral can depress immune function. Moreover, chances are that grocery store produce has

Mineral-Depleted Soil: Modern-Day Health Disaster

For centuries farmers put manure, seaweed or compost back into the soil, thereby enriching it with minerals and microflora that are routinely consumed by earlier crops. Make no mistake, if it isn't in the soil, it won't get into the fruit or vegetable and consequently won't supply your body. A mineral-deficient person can suffer from diminished immunity. In other words, a lack of selenium, magnesium, iron and zinc, amongst other minerals can impair immune response. The way that minerals, vitamins and other nutrients interact profoundly determines cellular immune mechanisms. I don't know about you, but I know very few people who grow their own mineral-rich foods. If they don't take the right supplements, they are probably low in certain minerals. Consequently, they may be at an increased risk of disease.

been chemically grown, treated with pesticides and herbicides, and artificially ripened with gases.

Living with Poisons That Exhaust Immunity

The various and sundry poisons we routinely live with cause everything from low sperm counts to lung disorders. A recent report published in *Environmental Pollution and Neuroimmunology* stated that the combined influence of various factors (chemical agents, radiation, stress, etc.) may lead to immune deficiency in the form of respiratory and inflammatory disease.

Hundreds of other studies show that exposure to toxic chemicals impairs immune defenses. Each and every day our bodies are bombarded with pollutants in the form of industrial chemicals and pesticides, synthetic hormonal imposters found in plastics, and noxious gases released in the atmosphere. To illustrate the gravity of this threat, researchers report there are between three hundred and five hundred toxins that inhabit human tissue, most of which didn't exist fifty years ago. Since the 1940s, our systems have been exposed to thousands of new chemicals that have found their way into not only our foods, but our air and water supplies as well.

Clearly, carbon monoxide, insecticides, chemical fumes and aluminum ingestion can wreak havoc with brain chemistry. In addition, rising infertility rates among women and declining sperm counts in men are attributed to the presence of heavy metals in seafood and a whole host of other chemical poisons. To make matters worse, RDAs (recommended daily allowances) of vitamins and minerals were never set up to deal with the array of mental and physical stressors that inhabit our environment.

Here's something else to ponder—perhaps the reason so many of us feel lousy day after day without any apparent

Pesticides Are Immuno-Toxic

Studies which involved the National Institutes of Health and the World Health Organization found that mortality rates from common infectious diseases may be caused in part by exposure to pesticides. Scientists reported that common pesticides also increase a person's risk of developing cancer by breaking down the immune system's surveillance system. They also found that infants, children and the elderly are at the greatest risk for what they referred to as "chemically induced immune suppression." Researchers found that 80 percent of children in the agricultural districts of areas where pesticides were used extensively had abnormal immune function. Children from those areas were three times more likely to have infectious diseases of the digestive tract, and from two to five times more likely to have infectious diseases of the respiratory tract. Moreover, people who worked in pesticide factories and on farms also showed elevated rates of infectious diseases. Study findings were so compelling that some experts called for a large-scale research program to establish a link between pesticides and immune system damage.

reason is that our cellular defense armies have to continually address the threat of scores of foreign invaders. The constant barrage of toxins, stress and microbes overworks our immune system, which usually attempts to meet the challenge without adequate weapons or reinforcements (nutrients, rest, etc.). The result—unexplained fatigue, low endurance and poor disease resistance.

Athletic Endurance and Glyconutrients

An article in the May 1999 issue of *Muscle & Fitness Magazine* entitled "What Can Glyconutrients Do for You?" reported that by boosting maximum immune responses, glyconutrients help to avoid the immune breakdown often seen after intense training.

In addition, dangerous free radicals are formed at a more rapid rate when we exercise. It is thought that by avoiding the severity of these internal breakdowns, gains in lean body mass may be enhanced or better maintained. It is also thought that glyconutrient supplementation may increase the efficiency of an athletic workout, so less exercise might render the same effect as more.

The Impact of Stress on Immune Function

I have to laugh every time a woman tells me that her doctor advises her to avoid stress. Short of entering a convent, a woman cannot completely avoid stress. Most women continually deal with stressors of all kinds. What most of them don't know, however, is that unmanaged, chronic stress can put them at increased risk for diseases of all kinds, including cancer. Someone once said that the human body was designed to resist an infinite number of changes and attacks brought about by its environment. One of the secrets of maintaining good health depends on our ability to make appropriate adjustments to changing stressors on the body. One thing is certain, continual emotional stress impairs the immune system (among other things). Personally, I describe stress as the silent killer of our time.

Chronic stress can substantially raise your susceptibility to diseases of all kinds. Researchers compared twenty-five parents of children who had cancer with twenty-five parents of healthy children. Naturally, the parents with sick children reported more psychological distress than the control group. But even more distressing is the fact that the hormones that turn on immune response were inhibited in this group.

One study of interest found that psychological stressors suppressed immune function in people who were sensitive to stress. In other words, if your heart rate and blood pressure go up in stressful situations, your immune efficiency is also likely to be negatively affected. Why? Because you release more epinephrine and norepinephrine when you get stressed, and those hormones suppress the action of natural killer cells. When your immune system is suppressed, latent viruses that have been dormant can emerge, triggering an attack of common viruses like herpes simplex or shingles. When you experience stress, your catecholamine levels go up. Consequently, immune cells become impaired.

Another very telling study found that peptic ulcers and ulcerative colitis occur twice as often in air traffic controllers as compared to civilian copilots, and the rate was even higher among air traffic controllers who worked at high-stress airports. Of particular interest is that a bacteria called H. pylori can cause stomach ulcers by breaking down the protective lining of the stomach. What this implies is that stress alone may not be the actual cause of an ulcer—but because stress in some people breaks down immunity, the H. pylori bacteria is allowed to flourish.

Stress can also make you more prone to viral infections. One study found that test subjects who became stressed showed a 25 percent increase in infection rates, and their incidence of colds almost doubled. Likewise, other studies reveal that students have a higher risk of mononucleosis during exams. I can tell you from personal experience that an immune breakdown can also occur after prolonged periods of stress—a kind of post-traumatic weakening of immune defenses. My daughter will inevitably come down with a serious sore throat after a stressful time in her life has ended. Studies support this phenomena. For example people get colds and flu more often on weekends after a busy work week. Of equal interest, test animals subjected to stress developed stomach ulcers during the time they actually rested and appeared to recover from the stress. Unquestionably, emotional stress also puts you at risk for disorders like allergic reactions, autoimmune disease, cardiovascular disease, and infectious and rheumatologic illnesses. Several other studies show that people who lose their spouse heal at slower rates than those who are not grieving. Moreover, other trials indicate that women who sustain prolonged periods of stress can be more prone to developing breast cancer in the future. Stress also releases histamines, which can trigger inflammatory reactions including asthma. Stress increases the risk for diabetes mellitus because it impacts insulin requirements and use. There is no question that chronic stress also contributes to the accumulation of plaque in the arteries, which raises your risk of angina and heart attacks.

Warning signs of a stress overload are many, and they vary widely from person to person. They include:

- insomnia
- nervousness and anxiety
- difficulty concentrating
- irritability
- fatigue
- headaches
- digestion problems
- depression
- weight loss or gain
- generalized muscle aches or back spasms

- panic attacks
- sudden rise in blood pressure
- breathlessness
- unexplained hot flashes

One of the most interesting studies I have run across reported that corticotropin-releasing hormone (CRH), which can be oversecreted during times of stress, impacts the immune system by affecting the action of the peripheral (immune) system. The chemical by-products of stress were found to selectively suppress cellular immunity. Of equal interest, people with major depression have lower serum tryptophan levels, which have been found to indicate an aggravated inflammatory response by the immune system—a finding that might explain why depression has been linked to unexplained aches and pains.

Antibiotic Resistance and "Super Bugs"

Hippocrates once said that "Natural forces within us are the true healers of disease." His comment seems particularly appropriate today. We've all shuddered at the thought of flesh-eating bacteria or smart strains of strep that can out-wit powerful drugs. Unfortunately, due to the overprescription of antibiotic drugs in this country, these super bugs are a reality. Once considered miracle drugs, antibiotic abuse is now a major health threat worldwide. Bacteria are now outwitting potent antibiotics creating the risk of global infections that won't respond to the best of the high-tech drugs. Richard Besser, M.D., of the CDC's (Center for Disease Control) respiratory disease branch has said, "Bacterial resistance to antibiotics is a growing public health threat to the United States."

In 1928, Alexander Fleming, a Scottish scientist discovered the first antibiotic. Subsequently, antibiotics became widely available during the 1940s. In the early 1950s, two million pounds of antibiotics were produced in the United States. Today that figure tops fifty million pounds. An antibiotic works by either killing bacteria or by inhibiting its growth. Statistics tell us that we consume well over 100 million doses of antibiotics every year. And 20 percent to 50 percent of that amount is considered unnecessary.

A Sobering Announcement

On June 12, 2000 in a press release, the World Health Organization announced that almost all major infectious diseases are slowly becoming resistant to existing medicines. The Centers for Disease Control and Prevention estimates that about 100 million courses of antibiotics are provided by

Antimicrobials and Incurable Germs

In April of 2003, the Journal of Clinical Microbiology published a study finding a number of antibiotic-resistant *Staphylococcus aureus* organisms in the blood samples of a patient who underwent extensive vancomycin chemotherapy for another infection. To put it another way, the cure created "incurable" germs. Similarly, another recent study discovered that the use of antimicrobials in food production has been associated with drug resistance in food-borne pathogens such as salmonella and campylobacter. They found that patients infected with multi-drug-resistant strains had a tendency towards higher mortality than patients infected with non-multi-resistant strains.

More Tips for Immune Building and Preventing Contagious Infections

- Wash your hands regularly.
- Take a multiple vitamin and mineral supplement that contains vitamin C, vitamin E, selenium, zinc, and beta-carotene for thymus (immune master gland) support.
- Get plenty of rest and sleep.
- Avoid white sugar.
- Drink alcohol in moderation.
- Don't smoke.
- Exercise.
- Control stress.
- Cover your mouth and nose for every cough and sneeze.
- Use a high efficiency home air purifier.
- Avoid misusing antibiotics including antibacterial soaps.
- Microwave dishrags and sponges for two minutes to kill germs.

medical doctors each year, many of which are for colds, coughs and other viral infections that don't respond to these medicines. The CDC recommends that everyone only use antibiotics when they are necessary.

It is also important to slow antibiotic use in farming to control bacterial infections. While the treatment may work, antibiotic residues can linger on the fruit causing the future development of resistant bacteria. Using antibiotics in livestock is also a concern. Not only does it encourage the evolution of super bugs, it gets into the human body as well.

The Predictions Are Grim

Antibiotics are only effective against bacteria and are completely useless against the viruses that cause the common cold, sinusitis, flu and some sore throats. Antibiotic abuse has transformed what were curable germs into new antibiotic-resistant bacteria. While antibiotics are certainly warranted for serious infections, the plant kingdom also provides herbal bug zappers that fortify our immune systems to successfully defeat infectious invaders. Before penicillin was discovered, herbs like echinacea were readily prescribed for infections by eclectic physicians of the late nineteenth century.

Tips to Lessen Antibiotic Resistance

- Wash raw fruit and vegetables thoroughly to clear off bacteria and antibiotic residue.
- Always complete a full course of antibiotics no matter how good you may feel to ensure that all disease-causing bacteria is destroyed. Do not save any of the pills.
- Don't ask for antibiotics if you have a cold, flu or any other viral infection.
- Don't continually use antibiotic ointments or hand lotions and soaps that contain antibacterial agents on a daily basis.
- Eat organic produce, meat and eggs.
- Build up your immune defenses to better handle the threat of infectious disease.

Are Hidden Infections to Blame for Unexplained Diseases and Disorders?

Scientists are discovering that diseases once thought to be unrelated to infectious invaders are really caused by microorganisms that either fail to trigger the proper immune response or overstimulate that response. One of the most fascinating studies came from researchers at the Department of Nutrition and Food Science at Wayne State University in Detroit. They reported in August 2002 that the storage of fat has been linked to the presence of a virus. Dutch scientists recently reported that chronic arthritis may have a bacterial connection. In fact, if you suffer from rheumatoid arthritis, which is considered an autoimmune disease, your disease may have been triggered by a prior infection that may have overstimulated immune responses, which in this situation needs suppressing. A German study published in the July 1993 issue of *Fertility and Sterility* reported that *E. coli* can actually adhere to sperm causing them to clump together.

In the August 2000 issue of the *American Journal of Medicine*, scientists reported that the hepatitis C virus can show up as a kidney infection or as heart disease. Last year, Italian researchers reported that the reason cholesterol deposits stick to the walls of arteries may be due to an infection not detected by the immune system that inflames blood vessel walls. The July 1999 issue of *Annals of Neurology* reported that a common bacteria called *Chlamydia pneumoniae* was present in all the patients tested in the study with multiple sclerosis. In addition 30 percent of people with MS also harbor the herpes virus.

In 1997, a group of scientists looked at a total of 135 people with epilepsy. More than 80 percent of these people had one or more abnormalities in their cellular immune defenses. An article in a 1994 issue of *Progress in Drug Research* reported that Alzheimer's disease may be linked to an abnormal antibody response to a portion of nerve cells in the brain.

Of equal importance, a chronic gum infection may even put your heart at risk. Some experts believe that pockets formed in gum disease are loaded with bacteria that can find its way into the bloodstream and eventually into the heart muscle itself. Of equal importance, hidden infections can compromise and weaken the immune system over time.

The Impact of Wholesale Vaccinations

Today, the typical American child receives over twenty vaccinations before the age of five. The widespread use of vaccinations over the last forty years has prompted some new controversy. Some health experts suggest that the alarming incidence of autism and ADHD, autoimmune diseases and various syndromes with no apparent cause over the last three decades is linked to the widespread use of vaccines. This notion has created unprecedented fear, which has been further fueled by the recall of contaminated vaccine serum or vaccines that contain mercury.

Concern has been so substantial that hearings on the subject were conducted by the U.S. Congress in 1999. The jury is still out. My own personal take on the issue is that while vaccinations have prevented countless deaths, they have exacted their own health toll. In other words, their benefits have come with a significant health price tag.

Allergic Reactions to Vaccine Components

Most parents don't know that children with allergies to eggs, antibiotics or chemicals like mercury can negatively react to vaccine ingredients. For example, polio vaccines and some MMR varieties contain a number of antibiotics. A moderately sensitive child may only react with a slight rash; however, if your child is allergic to antibiotics, that child may experience a severe reaction to being immunized. In addition, children who are allergic to egg protein may also have bad reactions to some MMR vaccines. Unfortunately, mercury is found in a number of vaccines and its inclusion has recently come under attack. There is a movement underway to remove all mercury from immunizing formulas. Some people believe that an intense reaction to mercury may be responsible for incidences of mental retardation or debility that occurs in some children postvaccination.

Dysfunctional Immunity: A Double-Edged Sword

In September of 2002, the Associated Press reported that people with weak immune systems were more likely to get seriously ill or die if they become infected with the West Nile virus. The article pointed out that if these people get the mosquito-transmitted virus, the likelihood of their recovery is less for them than for people with healthy immune systems. Interestingly, doctors found that eight of fifty-nine patients in an outbreak of the virus in New York City were known to have compromised immune systems. Consequently, experts recommended that anyone who has compromised immunity should pay extra attention to prevention. The real question here is this—is your immune system compromised and you don't know it? The following is a short list of factors that weaken immunity:

- free radicals
- alcohol
- tobacco
- dieting
- international travel
- eating disorders
- prescription drug side effects
- day care
- food additives
- aging

- lack of sleep
- poor digestion and elimination of waste
- consuming bad fats
- new viruses
- antibiotics

An Underactive or Overactive Immune System Equals Disease

If your immune system is too weak, you become susceptible to bacterial, viral, fungal and parasitic infections. If your
immune system is overactive, you become susceptible to
autoimmune diseases, where immune cells mistakenly attack
healthy human tissue; e.g., lupus, type I diabetes, rheumatoid
arthritis, psoriasis and Crohn's disease among others. Medical
science offers little in the way of a cure or effective treatment
for most of these diseases and many are escalating at an
alarming rate.

All disease states begin at the cellular level. In other words,
if our cells do not receive the right mix of nutrients, including
glyconutrients, they will not function optimally.
Consequently, our immune cells may

- fail to recognize, warn and mount an attack on invaders,
  which results in a higher risk of infection.
- transmit faulty signals, causing the immune system to
  mistake healthy tissue as a foreign invader called an antigen, which raises the risk of autoimmune diseases like
  rheumatoid arthritis and seasonal allergies.
- fail to recognize uncontrolled replicating mutated cells,
  which raises the risk of cancer.

Misunderstood Cells Equals Disease

Remember the "gossip game" we used to play as children? After the original message is whispered down the line from person to person, it becomes garbled and ends up hardly resembling its original form. Much in the same way, glycoprotein molecules that lack critical sugars can transmit all kinds of faulty information, or worse yet, say nothing at all. For example, cancer cells are allowed to grow unchecked because immune cells fail to recognize them. As a result, the usual command to mount an attack is never given. Having enough of the right "glycoforms" or sugar "coded" cells, keep cell messages accurate.

When the body has an assortment of glyconutrients to work with, glycoproteins can make more glycoforms. These cellular codes attach to the surface membranes of all kinds of cells. If the body is lacking in these sugars, the code can become corrupted. There is no question that people whose immune systems have been properly supported will deal with infection much more successfully.

Chapter Four

Humans as Plant Eaters

"I'm not a vegetarian because I love animals. I'm a vegetarian because I hate plants." –A.W. Brown

Glyconutrients come from plants—all kinds of plants. Before high-tech, genetically altered and synthetically replicated or refined foods hit our pantry shelves, humans ate a diet rich in plants, grains, tubers, seeds and nuts. Consequently, they continually fueled their bodies with vital plant sugars. Today, this is no longer the case. By and large, we don't eat the kinds of foods designed to optimize our immune defenses. To the contrary, the bulk of what we eat detracts from our body's ability to deal with health threats. The inevitable conclusion is that most of us lack the important dietary sugars we were meant to obtain through our consumption of plants.

According to the United States Department of Agriculture Health Freedom Resources, Inc. between 1900 and 1980,

- poultry consumption increased 350 percent.
- fresh apple consumption decreased 70 percent.
- fresh fruit consumption decreased 33 percent.
- fat and oil consumption increased 150 percent.

- margarine consumption increased 800 percent.
- corn syrup consumption increased 400 percent.
- sugar consumption increased 50 percent (the average person consumes 150 pounds of refined white sugar per year).
- cheese consumption increased 400 percent.
- soft drink consumption increased 300 percent.
- each person consumes 38 gallons of soft drinks annually (one fifth of our sugar intake is in soft drinks).

Just a side note—Americans eat an estimated seventy-five acres of pizza a day.

The Ways of Plant Eaters

Plant-eating animals like cows, sheep, and elephants subsist on herbs, grass, bark and leaves. Apes add fruits and nuts to the menu. The process of digesting these foods begins with an enzyme found in saliva called ptyalin. These animals have a set of special molars and they "chew their cud" so to speak with a side-to-side motion. Because they eat fibrous foods, their intestines are long as opposed to the shorter ones typically found in carnivorous animals.

Have you ever wondered if tigers and lions suffer from high cholesterol levels? After all, their diet is full of meat and saturated fats. Interestingly, meat-eating animals appear to have innate biological mechanisms that enable them to cope with so much meat and fat. On the other hand, in some experiments where animal fat was given to plant eating animals, those animals developed arteriosclerosis in a relatively short amount of time. The inevitable conclusion—plant eating creatures not only digest meat poorly, they also lack the ability to negate the harmful effects of a "meat-only" diet.

If you were to compare the human digestive system to that of the animal world, the species that we have the most in common with are the apes. We have similar teeth and digestive systems, but unlike the apes, we typically eat little fruit and nuts and way too much meat—something they would never do. Simple observation tells us that human beings were not designed to effectively digest meat. Modern-day research repeatedly confirms the fact that the consumption of animal fat has led to obesity, cancer, heart disease, gout and a whole myriad of degenerative diseases. By contrast, people who eat plenty of raw nuts, grains, fruits and vegetables have superior health and disease resistance.

Everything about our dental design, jaw structure and digestive processes supports the notion that we were meant to eat grains, legumes, nuts, fruits and vegetables and not meat. Our intestines are long, we cool our bodies through the process of sweating, and our saliva contains enzymes that expedite the digestion of grains. We humans are more predisposed to digest plants than meat.

- Carnivorous animals do not contain enzymes designed to initiate the digestion of starches. Human saliva contains these substances.
- Carnivorous animals secrete much more hydrochloric acid to digest skin, bones, cartilage and meat than humans do.
- The jaws of carnivorous animals move up and down to tear flesh and do not rotate from side to side to chew plants, etc.
- Carnivorous animals lap up liquids while humans drink liquid in by suction and simultaneous swallowing.

A Meaty Diet Can Be Murder

William C. Roberts, M.D., editor of *The American Journal of Cardiology*, said, "When we kill the animals to eat them, they end up killing us because their flesh, which contains cholesterol and saturated fat, was never intended for human beings, who are naturally herbivores." Many anthropologists agree that our early predecessors survived on a diet that primarily consisted of seeds, fruits and vegetables. Today, many of us eat meat at every meal—a habit that has profound consequences on our bodily functions and disease resistance.

Eating a diet high in meat and low in plants means that we will neglect to supply our bodies with the very nutrients designed to protect us from disease. Plants are our only source of essential sugars, not to mention scores of other valuable phytonutrients. Moreover, the saturated fats and cholesterol found in meat can be lethal to our cardiovascular systems. Dean Ornish, a well-known physician and author said, "I don't understand why asking people to eat a well-balanced vegetarian diet is considered drastic, while it is medically conservative to cut people open and put them on cholesterol-lowering drugs for the rest of their lives." So while we typically shop at our local grocery store for meat, eggs and milk, when it comes to immunity, we'd probably be better off if we chomped on tree leaves and plant stalks. In short, many health experts make a convincing argument that humans were not meant to eat flesh. William Castelli, another physician, put it this way, "Vegetarians have the best diet. They have the lowest rates of coronary disease of any group in the country. Some people scoff at vegetarians, but they have a fraction of our heart attack rate and they have only 40 percent of our cancer rate. They outlive other men by about six years now."

The Pros of Plant Eating

While many of us savor thick juicy steaks and mountains of barbecue ribs, gravitating to a diet higher in veggies, beans and fruits and lower in meat is certainly a good idea. In fact, Albert Einstein believed that nothing will benefit human health and increase chances for survival of life on Earth as much as the evolution to a vegetarian diet. Perhaps the evolution he refers to will require more of a dietary revolution to prompt most of us to eat meat sparingly or give it up altogether. Consider just a sampling of the health benefits of a vegetarian diet compared to the conventional American diet:

- Vegetarians are nearly 50 percent less likely to die from cancer than their meat-eating counterparts.
- Vegetarians have lower rates of heart disease and hypertension.
- Vegetarians have lower rates of diabetes.
- Vegetarians have lower rates of gallstones, kidney stones and osteoporosis.
- Vegetarians suffer less from PMS and menopausal symptoms.

The fact that fruits, vegetables and legumes are teeming with phytonutrients (plant nutrients) and fiber accounts for their extraordinary health benefits. When it comes to creating a super immune system, they are indispensable. Phytonutrients act as antioxidants; they positively alter estrogen metabolism; they prompt the destruction of malignant cells; they repair DNA damage caused by toxins like nicotine; they detoxify carcinogenic substances through enzymatic reactions; and they supply therapeutic sugars.

Live and Raw vs. Dead and Cooked

Someone once said that your cucumber should be well sliced, dressed with pepper and vinegar, and then thrown out. If you concur, you need to reconsider. Learning how to eat nutritiously revolves around the consumption of raw foods, and good habits begin in youth. Unfortunately, most of our kids have been raised to reach for the Twinkies or corn chips when they're hungry. How many kids do you know come home from school

Sweeping Your Cells

Cellular housecleaning—are you doing it? By now, we should all know that the better we can "round up" harmful free radicals, the better off our overall health and longevity will be. These dangerous oxidant compounds can actually deteriorate body tissue and are one reason that we age. Boosting the action of certain substances that houseclean our cells of these unstable molecules is a good thing indeed. One of the best cellular antioxidants in the body is called glutathione. Rola Barhoumi (a Ph.D. in Material Sciences) and her research team recently reported that glyconutrient supplementation increased the level of glutathione by 50 percent. It also prevented glutathione depletion in liver cells, where potentially harmful chemicals are detoxified. If we become low in glutathione, we can become vulnerable to degenerative diseases like diabetes and premature aging. This study suggests that taking a glyconutrient supplement containing the essential eight sugars helps protect our cells from free radical bombardment by boosting the action of glutathione, a powerful cell protectant. The essential eight also enhance tissue repair, help to control the appetite, and work to curb chemical addictions. The body's inability to use these sugars properly has also been linked to cystic fibrosis and anemia.

and snack on a tray of raw carrots, sliced apples, and celery sticks? On the contrary, when most kids are offered raw veggies, they turn up their noses. Virtually everything that passes their lips is either processed, baked, boiled or fried. In other words, the food (or something akin to it) that sustains most of our children is cooked, re-cooked, and overcooked.

In many cases, cooking transfers what was once a nutritious live food into a substance that bears little resemblance to anything produced by Mother Nature. How a diet deplorably low in raw foods impacts immunity could be the subject of another book, and what we're discussing is just the tip of the iceberg. Speaking of icebergs, when I ask young women if they eat enough raw veggies, I inevitably hear, "Oh yes, I eat tons of lettuce." A diet heavy in salads made from iceberg lettuce is far from nutritious.

Moreover, most of our meals are heavy on cooked foods and light on raw ones. Even when nutrient-rich, bioactive, fiber-filled food is overcooked, it is reduced to a completely different substance and its nutrient profile can be drastically altered. Vitamins, minerals and amino acids can be destroyed or altered depending on cooking temperature, method and time. Cooking processes like deep-fat frying can also create chemical changes in protein structures. These proteins can be more difficult to digest and have been implicated in everything from allergies to autoimmune diseases to cancer. Of equal importance, high cooking temperatures can create toxic chemicals.

You may be thinking, "I don't let my kids eat fried foods, and I never fry anything." Don't forget that corn chips, potato chips, curly cheese nips and other snack chips are usually fried. The current controversy over the health risks of Oreo cookies for kids is based on its content of trans-fats. These fats are often found in margarine and are created when liquid fats are artificially converted into solid ones. They are considered dangerous because they can cause cardiovascular disease by creating arteriosclerosis. Not only are our kids neglecting to eat food that contain glyconutrients, they are subsisting on edibles that can make them sick and fat.

Cooked Foods: The Enzyme Drought

An enzyme is one of the most remarkable structures found in nature. It jump-starts thousands of chemical reactions that sustain life. In order to digest properly and assimilate nutrients, we need to consume foods that contain enzymes. Unfortunately, enzymes present in raw foods are destroyed at most cooking temperatures. Many health experts believe that eating enzyme-lacking food stresses the pancreas and other organs and strains the immune system. As a result of continually consuming "dead" foods, body systems become stressed, poor digestion results and health consequences may run the full gamut: from chronic fatigue to autoimmune disease to fibromyalgia.

One theory behind this immune breakdown is based on the fact that after eating a cooked meal, white blood cells migrate to the digestive tract, leaving the rest of the body more vulnerable. This notion is based on the idea that cooked food is perceived as a foreign substance by the immune system. To make matters worse, cooked meat can change the makeup of intestinal flora causing a condition called intestinal toxemia, which can cause colitis, infections, yeast proliferation, etc. You can imagine what kind of havoc having a toxic waste dump wreaks on the immune system. In short, raw fresh foods provide our intestinal system with vital enzymes that properly breakdown food molecules. In addition, the high fiber content of such foods "sweeps" the colon, keeping it healthy and toned.

American Sources of Natural Gas

Eating a diet low in fruits and vegetables, fiber and high in sugar, fat and meat can create tummy troubles characterized by bouts with bloating and painful indigestion. While the simple elimination of gas after eating is the normal end-result (no

User-Friendly Bowel Bugs

Billions of beneficial or "friendly" bacteria reside in the colon. If the environment of the bowel remains hospitable, these bacteria multiply and maintain desirable numbers. These beneficial microorganisms synthesize vitamins, balance the acid/alkaline levels of the colon, assist in digestion, and fight infection. Similarly, most people chomping on cheeseburgers for lunch have no idea that the type of intestinal bacteria created in their colon depends on what they choose to eat. Many health experts emphasize that a diet high in meat creates bowel putrefaction and the formation of undesirable bacteria whose presence can cause bad breath, flatulence and recurring illnesses of all kinds.

Keep in mind that antibiotic therapy also kills friendly flora. In fact, new studies suggest that children who undergo repeated antibiotic therapy for earaches can develop a deranged form of intestinal bacteria that can promote the formation of yeast infections, which may affect behavior and learning. Any child who has taken antibiotics should be given an acidophilus supplement for at least three months to restore friendly bacteria.

Lactobacteria keep candida (yeast) in check. A chronic yeast infection creates continual stress on the immune system and predisposes a person to a variety of symptoms and ailments. Acidophilus supplements help to restore beneficial flora in the colon. Take one half teaspoon of acidophilus powder twice a day or use liquid supplements as directed first thing in the morning.

pun intended) of digestion, painful stomach cramping and bloating is not. Due to a poor choice of food (cooked and highly refined), the process of turning food into energy is a painful one for many Americans, and the problem affects all age groups. Colicky babies and school-aged kids with indigestion and gas abound.

How can something as natural as eating cause so much distress? Constipation, stress, lactose intolerance, smoking, and even antibiotic therapy can cripple digestive mechanisms so food fails to be broken down properly. Of equal importance, our digestive system was never designed to process the glut of sugary cold cereal, greasy potato chips, loads of processed cheese and incredible amounts of red meat. Consequently, eating makes a lot of people feel sick. Bloating, stomach cramps, diarrhea, nausea, fatigue and headaches are frequently the result of eating a meal.

I read once that pioneers who had to survive a winter on the plains were restricted to a diet of only wild game. Because of snow cover there were no weeds, plants or berries to harvest. After a few weeks, they became violently ill and instinctively knew that their "meat-only" diet was causing severe intestinal distress that could be fatal. Written journals of the event record that what happened next was divinely inspired. They were prompted to chip bark off of pine trees, boil it and drink the decoction. To make a long story short, the phytonutrients and glyconutrients contained in the bark saved their lives.

Paradise Lost

While we don't want to regress to the days of covered wagons, the future of our victory over disease may depend on looking back to the past. Clearly, the notion that glyconutrients may lessen the risk of, or even prevent scores of, diseases was known by ancient herbalists, who recognized plants, barks, and seeds that stimulated healing and wellness. Consider that much of what ancient medical practitioners prescribed has been validated by modern science. For example, Greek and Roman physicians used liver extracts to treat poor eyesight. Today we know that liver is rich in vitamin A, which prevents the development of night blindness. The same correlation applies to vitamin C depletion and scurvy, low iron levels and anemia, and a thiamin deficiency and diseases like beriberi.

During the 1940s, vitamin D was added to milk to help prevent childhood rickets, a devastating disease that deformed the bones of countless children. While the disease has virtually disappeared, vitamin D deficiency still plagues many middle-aged and older adults, contributing to the loss of bone (osteoporosis). Likewise, iodine has been routinely added to salt since 1930 to prevent goiter (an enlargement of the thyroid gland). The widespread availability of iodized salt has all but eliminated the disorder.

For over fifty years, white flour, cornmeal, and white rice have been enriched with three B vitamins: thiamin, riboflavin and niacin, along with the mineral iron. In 1998, folic acid was also added. The human body must have a continual supply of proteins, carbohydrates and fats to maintain its health. Clearly, our present-day eating patterns are alarmingly deficient in plants and whole grains. At this writing, glyconutrients have taken their place as the newest missing link in our nutrition chain. Like these other nutrients, it's only a matter of time before their supplementation will be considered essential to good health.

Chapter Five

The Saccharide Solution

"Take care of your body. It's the only place you have to live."

Jim Rohn

Until recently, the marvelous workings of beneficial saccharides have been minimized, overlooked or completely neglected by biochemists who thought they understood how cells work. Actually, Mother Nature provides glyconutrients in an infant's first meal, which explains why breast milk is such an extraordinary food.

Baby Your Baby: It Starts with the First Meal

I can remember when doctors discouraged women from breastfeeding and touted the superiority of commercial cow's milk formulas. What a health tragedy! That trend caused untold milk allergies, digestive woes, lower disease resistance and higher rates of sudden infant death syndrome for scores of children who are now adults. Thankfully, the tide has turned, although I believe that the profound merits of breast feeding are not publicized enough.

Human breast milk is loaded with an enormous variety of sugars. In and of itself, that fact supports the notion that the human body requires many different kinds of sugars to develop and thrive. Unfortunately, commercially produced baby formulas don't provide the same array of sugars found in breast milk. These beneficial saccharides were designed to not only keep a baby's immune defenses sharp, but to prevent allergies and infections while simultaneously ensuring proper brain development. Breast milk is a veritable immune potion; and while we understand that it transfers the mother's immune memory cells (antibodies) to her offspring, no one fully appreciates the profound role its sugar array plays in human development and survival.

As mentioned earlier, when certain sugars combine with protein molecules, a glycoprotein is born. These compounds are found on cell surfaces and have a diverse job description. They help maintain cell integrity and provide specific cellular signatures, so the immune system can recognize invaders and round up the troops on demand. To illustrate how a subtle change in their structure can produce profound effects, consider the fact that your particular blood type is determined by the sugar component of glycoproteins found in your blood serum.

A study published in a 1998 issue of *Biological Neonate* reported that several different glycoproteins found in breast milk can protect breast-fed babies against infection by microorganisms. The report explained that these proteins actually bind to bugs like *E. coli* and rotaviruses and mark them for destruction. In addition, the tests revealed that these sugar compounds actually inhibit the binding of the HIV virus to a host cell. Their conclusion—breast milk glycoproteins provide protection against several disease-causing organisms and the toxins they produce.

The primary sugar found in breast milk is lactose, but thirty or more oligosaccharides (complex sugars) are also present.

Protection from Infection

A recent study in *Biology of the Neonate* reported that components in human breast milk can protect breast-fed infants against microbial invasion. Four biochemicals were specifically pertinent to this protection: mucin, which inhibits the binding of *E. coli* to host cells; lactadherin, which prevents rotavirus-induced infection; glycoaminoglycans, which inhibit binding of HIV host cells; and oligosaccharides, which provide protection against several infectious agents and their toxins.

Among these are neuraminyloligosaccharides, mannose and fucose—sugars that keep breast-fed babies more resistant than their bottle-fed counterparts. These glycoproteins are also found in colostrum (the first milk), which is rich in antibodies whose molecules are constructed with sugar components.

Breast-Feeding and Future Disease Prevention

Studies indicate that the incidence of eczema and asthma in young children who were breast-fed was five times less frequent than in children who were fed formula. And the benefits of breast-feeding to prevent diarrhea and ear infections may last well past infancy. The sugars found in breast milk are created when an enzymatic reaction causes them to attach to galactose. In the case of intestinal infections, these sugars appear to protect breast-fed babies from gastrointestinal infections when glyconutrients prevent infectious organisms from sticking to intestinal cells. Breast milk isn't only rich in glycoproteins, it also contains an impressive array of other sugar-coated compounds that impact the inflammatory response and other immune mechanisms. It's no secret that breast-feeding babies is tantamount to their ability to resist and fight infection. In fact, international health organizations predict that if more women breast-fed their infants, deaths from upper respiratory and intestinal infections would dramatically decrease.

Providing the Right Cellular "Chatter"

Virtually every body function depends on the ability of cells to transfer data to each other. The "Ps and Qs" of this data are encoded in glycoproteins, which, as we mentioned, can be comprised of various sugars. In addition, glycolipids (fats) can perform similar functions. Proper cellular communication takes place because the "gridwork" found on cells' surfaces is in good working order. This information transfer occurs simultaneously throughout the body at many thousands of times per second. Try to imagine what would happen if the messages become corrupted or are missing altogether. Picture a poorly edited movie that jumps and skips from scene to scene, making it impossible to piece together a coherent plot. Sufficient evidence now exists to back the notion that when the body is deficient in certain saccharides or carbohydrates, cells miscommunicate, thereby initiating the development of disease.

"Sugar-Coded" Messenger Molecules

The status of our health depends on the ability of our cells to talk to each other. Virtually every body process that works to protect and heal us involves certain intercellular transmissions. These coded messages control everything from wound healing to cancer cell destruction. In fact, as mentioned earlier, the differences between the blood types A, O and B boils down to a subtle change in the individual glyconutrient profile of blood cells.

In the past, it was thought that proteins supplied cells with these codes. Just a few years ago, however, scientists discovered that certain sugar molecules bonded with proteins and determined how a cell communicates with its neighbor. The health implications of this discovery cannot be overestimated.

Sugar and protein molecules form chains that link together and pass on chemical codes that initiate either bad or good reactions in the body. Proteins also give sugars a "ride" and help to transport them throughout the body. Adding the right mix of sugars to the body boosts "cellular conversations," thereby enhancing the very reactions to restore health. "Chatty" cells make for optimal wellness.

Cellular Hieroglyphics

That tiny, seemingly insignificant lining (membrane) that surrounds each cell actually plays an enormous role in maintaining wellness. The condition of the cell membrane determines how efficiently cells can transmit and translate info. Glycoforming the cell surface with certain sugars is thought to maximize its ability to "talk" to its cellular neighbor. Think of glycoforms as cellular "words." If our cells fail to send the right signals or, even worse, transmit faulty information, disease can result.

For example, cells need to warn other cells when invaders enter the body and send for reinforcements in times of crisis. There are over two hundred monosaccharides found in nature and a minimum of eight are considered vital to efficient cell-to-cell talk. When this communication works as it should, the body fights off infectious invaders more effectively, healing is enhanced, and cellular detoxification is improved.

Unlike using too many antibiotics, which kills the good bacteria along with the bad, keeping the body supplied with glyconutrients boosts killer cell production safely, so only the bad guys get it.

Research suggests that few of us are getting an adequate supply of these plant sugars through our diets. In addition, experts believe that many of us fail to synthesize them properly. Typically, we obtain only two of the eight sugars we've discussed from dietary sources. Our bodies must then work to manufacture the other six or obtain them through product supplementation. While we have the ability to produce some glyconutrients, to do so requires complex chemical pathways. The harmful effects of stress, toxins, poor nutrition and genetic abnormalities in our metabolism can inhibit this conversion or require that it occur at a faster-than-normal rate. Consequently, the number and structure of our glycoproteins may be impaired. Hence, we contract disease.

Fooling Sugar-Coated Bacteria

It's important to know that a whole host of disease-causing organisms make use of sugar molecules to invade human host cells. The idea behind "sugar-coated" drugs or natural sugar supplements is that they mimic receptor sugars on host cells, thereby fooling invader cells. In other words, the germs bind to the imposter molecules rather than to human cells. In so doing, the extent or duration of the infection is decreased.

In addition, because bacterial microbes have the advantage of also having a sugar coating that protects them from destruction, we need specially equipped immune agents to tag and destroy them. Fortunately, our clever immune systems make marvelous entities called antibodies. Antibodies bind to the tough, sugar-coated bacteria, making it possible for macrophages to attach and consume them. Without antibodies, the sugar-coated surface of a bacteria would actually repel macrophages, making it impossible to destroy them.

So, the more antibodies you have, the better your ability to fight bacterial infections. This may partly explain why young children are more susceptible to bacterial infections—their immune systems are immature and are still in the process of accruing antibodies.

The artificial stimulation of antibodies also brings up the question of what really happens when vaccines are introduced into the bodies of babies and toddlers. Unquestionably, the artificial stimulation of antibodies in the immune systems of children have saved countless lives. There is, however, a possible downside to early vaccinations, and the jury is still out. At this point, it's important to keep in mind that many vaccines are composed of polysaccharides. It's also important to understand that the antibodies that attach to the polysaccharide coat of bacteria belong to a category called IgG2 and IgG1. You may recall that gamma globulin shots used to be recommended for some people with weakened immunity—a substance that belongs to the IgG2 class.

The Antigen Factor

As we discussed earlier, all cells and infectious microorganisms carry surface "ID tags" called antigens, which stimulate the immune system to produce antibodies against them. Each of these individual molecular signatures tells our immune cells whether the microorganism is friend or foe. Amazingly, immune defense cells recognize and respond to thousands of antigens. However, many infectious agents routinely mutate, confusing our immune system. This phenomenon explains why we can catch multiple colds and flus over the course of time.

A Spoonful of Glyconutrients Helps the Medicine Go Down

Taking glyconutrients on a daily basis may be one of the most powerful ways to boost our defenses against disease. Continual supplementation can provide and augment desirable chemical actions that keep immune agents in tip-top shape. In today's health-threatening environment, we need to act before, not after, the fact. Unfortunately, the preventive approach to health flies in the face of the narrow-minded view of conventional medicine. Leo Galland, author of *Superimmunity for Kids*, puts it this way, "It's tragic that the tremendous power of science has not been placed at the disposal of a much older model that views the job of the healer as helping a person to restore harmony and balance."

Glyconutrient supplementation can help to correct an overactive immune system (autoimmune diseases), boost an underactive immune system (chronic or recurring infections) and keep the immune system in tip-top shape for exceptional disease prevention.

Scientific data strongly suggests that supplementation of these sugars is the only way to ensure that glycoproteins have what they absolutely need to function properly.

Having an enviable glycoprotein profile is what keeps our immune systems in great working condition by keeping cellular communication sharp and accurate. When the message breaks down, so do we. Regarding autoimmune diseases, which occur when immune cells get the wrong message, using glyconutrients as part of a daily supplemental plan may help to correct cellular codes. In short glyconutrient supplementation may fight, and more importantly, prevent viral, fungal and parasitic infections, autoimmune diseases, cancer and other bacterial and mycobacterial diseases, and neurological diseases.

Is Glyconutrient Supplementation Backed by Scientific Research?

Over twenty thousand studies have been conducted on individual glyconutrients and virtually all of them have positive outcomes. Research has proven that these sugars significantly contribute to immune function.

Studies confirm that these beneficial sugars can

- dramatically raise natural killer cell and macrophage count against infectious organisms
- activate immune T cell activity only when invaders or antigens are present
- decrease cell death in people suffering from chronic fatigue syndrome
- dramatically elevate disease resistance in weakened individuals
- act as antioxidant compounds that boost the collection of dangerous free radicals
- protect the body against toxin and pollutant exposure
- slow premature aging
- decrease inflammation in diseases like rheumatoid arthritis
- help immune cells recognize invaders due to a mutual "sugar exchange" of info
- enable cellular components to stick to each other initiating the right reactions

Scientists at the Glycobiology Institute at Oxford recently discovered that macrophages (the immune cells that eat invaders) have mannose receptors that activate immune attacks. Macrophages are also dramatically influenced by two other members of the essential eight sugars called fucose and N-acetylglucosamine.

Mounting scientific evidence backs the use of glyconutrients for both the prevention and treatment of illnesses that include fibromyalgia, chronic fatigue syndrome, osteoarthritis, lupus, candida and rheumatoid arthritis. Medical science offers little in terms of curing or even managing these diseases. Unfortunately, the drugs used to ease the symptoms of these diseases (anti-inflammatories, steroids, etc.) come with significant side effects. On the other hand, natural immune boosters are relatively nontoxic and work to address the root of the problem rather than its presenting symptoms.

Of equal importance, supplementing the body with these sugars not only boosts immune function, it also helps to modulate or normalize an overactive immune response. It does so at the cellular level, appearing to "recalibrate" cell-to-cell communication. It's all about restoring balance.

Adaptogenic Sugars: How They Compare to Pharmaceutical Drugs

Primitive ancient medical practitioners knew what we have to relearn today—that some plant compounds have a brain. In other words, when you take glyconutrients or other adaptogenic plant compounds, they enter the body and act according to need. They either kick in and prompt reactions that heal when you're sick or work through other pathways to prevent illness. Stated simply, they help the body adapt to its particular health challenge and environment. To put it another way—they initiate healing rather than just mask the symptoms of disease. No prescription high-tech drug can do that. Consuming glyconutrients does not treat disease directly. It does lots more than that—it enables the body to optimize its own functions and systems that promote healing and protection from within.

Chapter Six

Sugar-Rich, Immune-Boosting Plants

"There are no incurable diseases—only the lack of desire. There are no non-healing herbs—only the lack of knowledge."
—attributed to Chinese medicinal texts

Herbal medicine is nothing new. Virtually every culture on earth uses plants in medicinal applications. And, believe it or not, up until the turn of the twentieth century, herbs were still listed in the *Physician's Desk Reference*. Unfortunately, herbal remedies fell out of favor with the advent of drug manufacturing. The "modern" consensus is that synthetic drug compounds are more effective than plant-based therapies. Today, our widespread dependency on prescription drugs and their potential drawbacks has stimulated a new American herbal renaissance. Make no mistake—one of the main reasons so many of these botanicals fight disease is their glyconutrient content. Keep in mind that many pharmaceutical drugs use natural plant compounds as the basis for their chemical design. As we mentioned earlier, new glycodrugs are currently in the research stage because experts recognize their enormous therapeutic potential.

Herbs and Synthetic Drugs

Unlike synthetic drugs, herbs rich in glyconutrients provide a complete and synergistic array of compounds that enhance each person's ability to fight and protect against disease. Moreover, plant compounds are usually well tolerated in the human body because they are perceived as familiar chemicals. By contrast, synthetic drugs come with significant side effects because the body reacts to them as foreign substances—the price we commonly pay for rapid symptom management. It's important to remember that, just like anything in nature, herbs work more slowly than most drugs.

Plants with Medicinal Punch

As mentioned earlier, it is the sugar portion of both our immune cells and invading organisms that transfer vital messages—messages that determine whether we get sick or not, or how long we stay that way. Herbal practitioners have known for millennia that plants rich in these special sugars can spike immune chain reactions to better combat infections and boost healing.

Hundreds of plants contain compounds called "glycosides" or sugar derivatives. Recently these extraordinary compounds have generated a great deal of attention because they possess a variety of desirable properties. Be assured that most of the herbs designated as powerful immune complements are full of complex sugars called polysaccharides, which stimulate desirable immune activity.

Polysaccharide Prowess

Polysaccharides are more complex (long-chained) sugar

molecules that contain multiple saccharide links. And while they're not as soluble as simple sugars, they are considered more stable. Some polysaccharides are digestible and others are not. For example, starch and dextrin are easily broken down in the body, while cellulose and hemicelluloses are not digested and pass through the intestinal tract unchanged.

While ancient practitioners were unaware of their chemical profile, they knew that certain botanicals actively fought infections. Today, we can identify polysaccharide-rich plants and their immune-boosting actions and clearly, they are nothing less than remarkable.

Polysaccharides Potentiate Immune Pathways

When an infectious invader enters the human body, vital immune defense mechanisms use polysaccharides to

- boost phagocytosis (the eating of the bad guys by the good guys).
- increase the gathering of phagocytes (germ-eating cells) to foreign cells.
- enhance the destruction of microbes by bursting their cell walls.
- stimulate desirable substances (interferon, interleukin, etc.) that fight tumors, bacteria, viruses and fungi.
- inactivate or disable certain viruses by inhibiting their replication.
- defend against dangerous bacterial poisons.
- support the inflammatory process, which increases the ability of phagocytes to rush more effectively to areas of infection.
- defend against dangerous bacterial poisons.
- support the inflammatory process which increases the ability of phagocytes to rush more effectively to areas of infection.
- suppress inflammation when appropriate.

Aloe Vera

Aloe vera is a tried-and-true plant remedy backed by scores of scientific studies that support its use (both internally and externally). Aloe has been used for everything from detoxification, tissue healing and regeneration, intestinal disorders, joint and muscle pain, inflammation and infections of all kind. For our purposes, it's important to know that you can judge a good source of aloe by its polysaccharide content.

One reason that aloe products should be kept in dark containers at cool temperatures is to slow the action of an enzyme called cellulase, which breaks down polysaccharides—a process that can begin shortly after harvesting aloe vera leaves. In addition, be aware that using alcohol-processed aloe vera products can also destroy these fragile sugar molecules. Most of the polysaccharides and therapeutic agents found in aloe are located in the jelly-like substance found in the leaf. Aloe vera gel contains two important sugars: glucomannan and mannose—a duo that kicks immune function up a notch.

Mighty Mannose

Mannose-6 phosphate is the primary sugar constituent of aloe vera extract and it stimulates a number of desirable biological changes. Mannose prompts anti-inflammatory activity and tissue regeneration. It also activates something called insulin-like growth factor receptors, which is a good thing. Mannose also stimulates fibroblasts to make more collagen and proteoglycans, which means better and faster healing from burns, cuts, etc. It also appears to lessen pain and increase the strength and integrity of skin cells.

Aloeride: New Kid on the Block

In February 2001, the *Journal of Agriculture and Food Chemistry* reported the discovery of a compound called aloeride (a new polysaccharide extracted from the juice of the aloe vera leaf). This compound contains glucose, galactose, mannose and another sugar called arabinose and has been called a powerful immune booster. The discovery illustrates the notion that even now, we continue to uncover new sugars in plant sources that contribute to human health.

Aloe's Acemannan

Acetylated mannose, also known as acemannan, is a marvelous bioactive sugar component found in aloe vera. This glyconutrient has been shown to be a powerful, effective immune stimulant that fights viruses that cause flu, measles, and even the early stages of AIDS. While acemannan contributes to aloe's remarkable healing properties, its impact on immune pathways is equally impressive. In a variety of scientific trials, acemannan significantly boosted the number and effectiveness of T lymphocytes, which go after microbial invaders. In addition, acemannan has significant antitumor actions. In fact, for this reason, aloe has been effectively used to treat some veterinary cancers (sarcoma specifically) and is under investigation as a possible cancer therapy in humans. Other sugars found in aloe include arabinose, cellulose, galactose and xylose.

Echinacea purpurea

Considered a star among herbal immune boosters, echinacea is rich in polysaccharides and a natural antibiotic-like chemical called inulin. Inulin stimulates and mobilizes white blood cells into areas of infection, helping to better eradicate a broad range of bacteria, viruses, and other microorganisms. Echinacea's most powerful immune-boosting polysaccharides are called heteroglycans, and they contain a variety of therapeutic sugars.

These compounds increase the germ-eating capacity of phagocytes and stimulate macrophages to produce an array of chemicals needed by the immune system. Some of these include interleukin-1, interleukin-6, and the tumor-necrosis factor alpha (causes tumors to self-destruct).

Echinacea Targets T Lymphocytes

A new study conducted by scientists at McGill University in Montreal, Canada showed that two weeks of supplementation with echinacea rejuvenated the production of immune killer cells even in animals of advanced age. Moreover, a University of Munich study showed that echinacea boosted production of infection-fighting T lymphocytes up to 30 percent more than standard immune-supportive drugs. That is a significant statistic. A dose of thirty drops of echinacea extract taken daily for five days resulted in a whopping 120 percent increase in the white blood cells that eat viral invaders for lunch.

Ideally, it's best to use echinacea in two-week intervals as a preventive agent or to take it during the initial stages of an infection. If you're already sick, maximum stimulation from echinacea occurs between three to six days after the first dose, so it needs to be taken at the first sign of an infection.

Medicinal Mushrooms

For millennia, a number of mushrooms (maitake, reishi, shiitake and coriolus among others) were used by Asian practitioners to prevent and fight disease. To illustrate, the reishi mushroom was traditionally referred to as the "mushroom of immortality." The glyconutrients in these fungi help the body repel invading microbes and even discourage the formation of tumors by fine tuning and fortifying natural immune defenses. In other words, they stimulate cell-mediated immunity by activating immune cells—so much so, that three anticancer drugs used in Japan have been extracted from compounds found in these mushrooms. In fact, an extract of the coriolus mushroom is one of the best-selling cancer drugs in Japan and Europe.

Mushroom's Glyconutrients

Finally recognized for their tremendous therapeutic value in this country, immune-friendly fungi work because they are rich in polysaccharide molecules. These mushroom sugars boost white blood cell numbers and their efficiency. Their sugar profile can not only enhance the destruction of invaders, but also can boost the postcellular collection of toxic waste materials. Interestingly, only fifty or so varieties of mushroom have this kind of medicinal prowess. While most people think of shiitake, maitake or reishi mushrooms as immune boosters, another one called *Cordyceps sinensis* is just as valuable.

Cordyceps Sinensis: Tri-Sugar Herbal Workhorse

Cordyceps sinensis is another highly esteemed Chinese mushroom, although some classify it as a parasitic fungi. The herb is available as a single supplement or is often included in immune-boosting formulas. Cordyceps is rich in glucose, galactose and mannose and activates a number of immune defenses by enhancing the production of interleukin-1 and 2, helper-T and natural killer cells. By so doing, it expands the capacity of the immune system to react and destroy infectious invaders, carcinogenic substances and malignant cells. It also has the innate ability to suppress an overactive immune system.

One of the main differences between synthetic drugs and glyconutrient-rich herbs is that nature's medicines can either rev up a weak immune system or suppress an overactive one. Recently, scientists have discovered that compounds found in the fungi *Cordyceps sinensis* may be effective in treating autoimmune diseases by suppressing inappropriate immune responses. In fact, the authors of the study concluded that due to its effectiveness, cordyceps should be investigated as a "pharmacologic intervention" for autoimmune disorders. Likewise, another study backed up these findings by reporting that cordyceps can prevent lupus attacks on the kidneys. Their findings: the therapeutic effect of cordyceps was markedly effective in twenty-six cases or 83.9 percent of test subjects treated. What these and other studies suggest is that cordyceps normalizes immune activity as needed.

In March of 2003, *Biotechnology Programs* published a study that discovered the production of an exopolysaccharide from a newly isolated cordyceps species. The implications: we are just beginning to scratch the surface when it comes to glyconutrients and how they really work. We do know that cordyceps stimulates T lymphocyte activity and has been successfully used to treat everything from hepatitis B to lupus.

Beta-glucans: Carbohydrate Powerhouses

Beta-glucans are a class of sugars found in medicinal mushrooms and other fungal plants such as astragalus. Beta-glucans are comprised of sugar chains that work to modulate the immune system. Their immune action is so dramatic that they are currently being investigated as a possible treatment for AIDS and cancer. Beta-glucans are also found in baker's yeast and in oat and barley bran.

In fact, eating oat bran lowers your cholesterol because of the action of these remarkable sugars. Of particular interest is the fact that beta-glucans have proven their ability to prolong life in cancer patients, fight massive infections in immune-compromised individuals, enhance recovery from radiation treatments, speed tissue regeneration in cuts and burns, and even prevent the onset of shock. These extraordinary polysaccharides also fortify the ability of antibodies to respond to invaders by increasing the memory capacity of T cells, so they can better gobble up germs and boost disease resistance.

The Sugars with a Brain

The beauty of beta-glucans and other therapeutic sugars is that they boost immune defenses on demand. In other words, beta-glucans have a brain. If you have an autoimmune disease, they don't put your immune system into overdrive—keeping your symptoms from getting worse. Of equal importance, one of the major drawbacks of chemotherapy is that white cells are killed along with cancer cells, putting a cancer patient at a heightened risk for infection. Beta-glucans help to keep white blood cell counts more elevated.

Another major advantage of taking beta-glucan supplements is that they are well absorbed and go to work rapidly. They can also be taken to prevent, rather than just treat disease. Beta-glucan supplements are recommended to treat anorexia, ulcers, liver disease, cancer, high cholesterol, and bacterial, viral and parasitic infections. There is some evidence that adding vitamin C to a beta-glucan supplement potentiates its absorption into the bloodstream. When shopping for a

Beta-glucans—Tumor Busters

A compelling study published in the November 2002 edition of *Cancer Immunology & Immunotherapy* reported that giving beta-glucans orally enhanced the action of antibodies that fight tumors. Beta-glucans were able to stimulate leukocyte CR3 activity, which means that tumor cells will be better destroyed. Moreover, this impressive effect worked regardless of the human tumor type, which includes neuroblastoma, melanoma, lymphoma and breast carcinoma. Scientists conducting the study concluded that, "Given the favorable efficacy and toxicity profile of oral beta-D-glucan treatment, the role of natural products that contain beta-glucan in cancer treatment as an enhancer of the effect of mAb therapy deserves further study." Another recent trial found that the sugar polymers known as beta-1,3-D-glucans exert potent effects on the immune system by stimulating antitumor and antimicrobial activity. How do they do that? By binding to receptors on macrophages (cells that eat the bad guys) and other white blood cells and activating them. The study emphasized that there is new evidence that an unknown beta-glucan receptor is present on macrophages, which provides new insights into how the innate immune system recognizes and benefits from beta-glucans.

beta-glucan supplement, look for a product that is standardized for 6 percent polysaccharides.

Lentinan: Fungal Superstar

While no one is suggesting that you snack on mold or wild mushrooms, another sugar metabolite found in certain therapeutic fungi called lentinan can also be called an immune wonder. So much so that it is referred to as an "immunomodulator" and has been used for centuries to treat cancer. Modern-day scientists have become fascinated with lentinan (better late than never). In fact, researchers have investigated the compound extensively, and scientists around the world laud its immune benefits.

What is lentinan? Technically, it's a beutral polysaccharide—an immune heavyweight that attacks cancer cells by empowering "immune potentiators." It does so by increasing the process by which immune effector cells reach maturity, so they can protect the body more efficiently. An effector cell describes an immune entity that coordinates with other immune defenders to eradicate disease organisms. Lentinan is found in a variety of medicinal mushrooms.

Arabinogalactan

Another impressive polysaccharide comes from the sap of various trees and plants. It's called arabinogalactan. Also known as gum sugar, this compound is readily found in a variety of vegetables and fruits, as well as in the immune-stimulating herb we call echinacea. Ironically, most gum sugars are used commercially only to improve and emulsify the texture of foods and cosmetics. Psyllium seed, a well-known and widely prescribed source of fiber for constipation also contains gum sugar.

Just this year, a study published in *Plant Molecular Biology* reported that arabinogalactan-proteins (AGPs) play an important role in cell-cell recognition, and programmed cell death (what keeps cells from growing into malignant tumors). Another recent study confirmed that these sugars positively affect the chemical nature of fecal matter, which can dramatically impact colon health by determining the kind of bacteria that inhabits the bowel. In addition, arabinogalactans have proven antiviral actions against hepatitis B. They also exert a multifaceted defense against all kinds of infectious organisms; and like beta-glucans, stimulate the action of lymphocytes, macrophages, white blood cells and cytokines—the best forces in our immune army. Gum sugars also fortify NK (natural killer) cells, which are programmed to seek and destroy viruses.

Pectins

Used to give jellies and jams their firmness, pectin comes from fruits like apples, pumpkins and tomatoes. Pectin is a form of fiber and has proven cholesterol-lowering properties. The fact that most of us fail to eat enough fruit once again supports the notion that we do not adequately obtain glyconutrients from our diets. In addition, one of the reasons a diet high in fruit is cancer protective is due, in part, to the glyconutrient content of fruit pectin. A 1997 report found in a well-known cancer journal revealed that apple pectin has definite anticancer effects in the colon. Another report published in the *Journal of Physiological Biochemistry* confirmed that the pectin in oranges and apples significantly decreased cholesterol levels in the liver.

It amazes some people that something as seemingly benign as pectins can exert so much immune muscle. An interesting study found in the January 2003 issue of *Microbiology Letter*, reported that pectin-oligosaccharides actually inhibit dangerous *E. coli* bacteria. They did it by blocking the toxicity of toxins produced from *Escherichia coli*. Interestingly the pectins that provided the most protection were those with the best oligosaccharide levels and resulted in 90–100 percent cell survival. Findings like these shed new light on the veracity of the old adage, "An apple a day keeps the doctor away."

Algaes

For hundreds of years, seaweed has enjoyed preferential status as a dietary staple in both Asian and Polynesian diets. As a food, many seaweeds contain more vitamin C than fruits like oranges. The notion that brown seaweeds like limu moui and sea plants like blue-green algae and spirulina have curative powers for human diseases is nothing new. Folk practitioners have used these plants to treat cuts, burns, sore throats, allergies, arthritis, bowel disorders, colds, flu, rashes, infections, tuberculosis, parasites, tumors and ulcers.

Today, the discovery of long-chain or complex polysaccharides in sea plants like limu moui helps explain their extraordinary curative powers. While all of the traditional medicinal uses for seaweeds have not been substantiated by medical research, what has been done confirms that marine algaes offer a myriad of remarkable health benefits. Unfortunately, North Americans have had little success cultivating a taste for sea vegetables.

Seaweed: A Remarkable Sugar-Rich Food

Statistically speaking, people who routinely eat seaweed dishes enjoy exceptional longevity and have a lower incidence of cancer compared to their Western counterparts. The inclusion of various types of brown seaweed in their diet is thought to be a major contributing factor to their impressive health statistics. Brown seaweed and other ocean plants contain a number of glyconutrients including fucose, mannose, galactose and xylose. One seaweed called laminaria even contains a substance that was recently discovered in Japan. It causes cancer cells to self-destruct and is called U-fucoidan (one of several polysaccharides found in brown seaweed). Fucoidans are a class of sulphated polysaccharides (large sugars with sulphate groups attached) that are widely dispersed in the seaweed cell wall. Japanese research found that when U-fucoidan was administered to cancer cells in a laboratory dish, they were virtually wiped out within seventy-two hours.

The process that withered the cancer cells away was self-induced, in that the DNA within each of them was broken down by digestive enzymes contained in the cells themselves. This process is called "apoptosis" and refers to cell self-destruction. Most normal, healthy cells automatically self-destruct when something goes wrong in their DNA. But sometimes free radicals and other outside influences block this natural process.

Polysaccharides called agars and carrageenans are also found in certain red seaweeds. These sugars have a wide range of properties and uses, and we routinely consume them everyday without knowing it. Carrageenans are used to keep chocolate milk smooth and homogenized. And agar gels are used in petri dishes to grow bacteria and add a smooth texture to desserts and jellies. Seaweed alginates are used in wound dressings, in keeping beer smooth and in cosmetic products. Agarose (derived from agar gels) is used to culture cells for DNA recognition.

Spirulina and Virus-Fighting Sugars

Spirulina belongs to a family of blue-green algaes rich in polysaccharides that enhance the reproduction of immune cells when the body is under attack. For this reason, spirulina

Brown Seaweed and Galactofucans

A new study found in *Carbohydrate Research* reported that sugars called "galactofucans" found in brown seaweed have impressive activity against herpes simplex virus 1 and 2 with no toxicity to healthy cells. Herpes, like other viral infections, is extremely difficult to get rid of. Interestingly, while brown seaweed has a variety of immune-supporting compounds, its sugar or carbohydrate biochemicals appear to be the most immune supportive. Scientists at the Institute of Marine Sciences of the University of North Carolina at Chapel Hill found that viral defense actions occurred in compounds that contain carbohydrate biochemicals, especially sulfated sugars.

supplements are often recommended to people with herpes simplex virus 1, cytomegalovirus, measles, mumps, influenza A and even HIV-1. All of these viral infections are resistant to most medications and are difficult to manage.

Spirulina sugars appear to inhibit the penetration of a virus into human host cells. Remember, viruses are microbial terrorists. They take healthy cells hostage, hijack their protein-making machinery, replicate themselves, and repeat the process in another cell. To make matters worse, some viruses are shape shifters, so our army of antibodies has a hard time keeping up. And viral invaders are opportunists. When we let our immune guard down (poor diet, sleep deprivation, stress, etc.) they move in.

Spirulina sugars have potent antiviral properties, and one of its polysaccharides called calcium spirulan (Ca-SP) is responsible in that it prevents viruses from replicating. Spirulina sugars can also help correct anemia, even when blood cells have been exposed to radiation. In addition, glycolipids (fats) found in spirulina called palmitic acid and linolenic acid are also good for controlling inflammation and have antitumor actions. One very interesting study found that spirulina polysaccharides actually inhibited the replication of malignant cells by disrupting their DNA functions.

Astragalus

Astragalus is another Chinese botanical rich in polysaccharides. Like many of the other plants we've been talking about, astragalus increases the action of microbe-eating cells. It also helps to transform T cells into helper cells to boost the digestion of dangerous microbes and invaders. Astragalus also speeds the production of interferon and the cellular clearing of toxins. Moreover, astragalus can increase the number of potentially harmful antibodies (IgA and IgG) in the blood. Of particular interest—in human and clinical trials, astragalus was able to significantly increase the survival rate of cancer patients who were on chemotherapy or radiation.

Anyone facing chemotherapy should become acquainted with astragalus. A very recent study found that astragalus supplementation enhanced the action of chemotherapy while it simultaneously protected healthy cells. Show me a drug that can do that? One hundred and twenty tumor patients were randomly divided into a treated group and a control group. Both groups were treated with chemotherapy, but the treated group received astragalus injections once a day for twenty-one days. Compared with the control group, the treated group showed a lower progression of cancer, less destruction of white blood cells and better overall counts of other immune cells and substances. They concluded that astragalus supplemented with chemotherapy could inhibit the development of malignant tumors, decrease the toxic-adverse effect of chemotherapy, elevate immune function and improve the quality of life in cancer patients.

Licorice

Licorice is an aromatic herb that has been used for millennia in the Mediterranean and Middle East as a medicinal agent. Along with an impressive array of actions, Licorice inhibits the chemical processes that leads to excessive inflammation in the body. What's more, licorice may also stimulate the production of antibodies, therefore boosting the body's resistance to viral and bacterial invaders. Licorice contains a compound called glycyrrhizinic acid, a sugar that is fifty times sweeter than white sugar. Upon hydrolysis, this glycoside loses its sweet taste and is converted to the aglycone glycyrrhetinic acid plus two molecules of glucuronic acid. This compound also has expectorant and antitussive properties used to either break up mucus or to increase its secretion depending on need. Glycyrrhizin also inhibits liver cell injury caused by exposure to toxic chemicals and is used in the treatment of chronic hepatitis and cirrhosis. It also inhibits the growth of several DNA and RNA viruses and is useful in inactivating herpes simplex virus particles irreversibly.

Black Pepper

If you like to pepper your food, now you have good reason. Black pepper contains some heavy-duty polysaccharides that include galactose, arabinose, galacturonic acid and rhamnose. Based on scientific testing, researchers have concluded that the sugars found in black pepper have a significant immune-fortifying effect. In fact, last year a study reported that polysaccharides from black pepper should be considered as a supplement for immune enhancement. Apparently, a compound called piperine, derived from black pepper, also increases blood levels of coenzyme Q10, an antioxidant that has a variety of valuable health benefits.

A Note on Yeast Polysaccharides

I remember when my grandmother made me take a teaspoon of brewer's yeast granules every day. She said it would keep the germs away. You know what? She was right. Yeast polysaccharides work to stimulate immune activities by providing support for the macrophages that eat germs for lunch. Case in point—for my husband, the only thing that worked to clear a case of boils caused by a staph infection was a brewer's yeast supplement.

In addition to their immune-stimulating properties, yeast polysaccharides also contribute to the regeneration of cells. Scientists have recently documented the antiviral properties of the sugars found in brewer's yeast on thirteen kinds of viruses. The report stated, "The result showed that this effect was remarkable on the infections with poliovirus III, adenovirus III, ECHO6 virus, enterovirus 71, vesicular stomatitis virus, herpesvirus I, II, Coxsackie A16 virus and Coxsackie B3 virus." Furthermore, the sugars found in brewer's yeast actually protected cells from being infected with the above viruses. Russian scientists also discovered that yeast sugars stimulate the activity of macrophages and the process by which they destroy pathogens (phagocytosis). Today, using brewer's yeast as a supplement is not as popular as in years past due to yeast sensitivities. Moreover, because candida infection is a major concern, if you have any sensitivity to yeast, then it's best to avoid brewer's yeast or supplements containing yeast.

Chapter Seven

Glyconutrients for Diabetes and Hypoglycemia

"Nature is capable of producing the most stunning effects with the smallest means." *–Henrich Heine*

You can't sugar coat the statistics. As the seventh leading cause of death in this country, over fifteen million people have diabetes. A shocking 798,000 new cases are diagnosed each year. Diabetes comes in two varieties: type I and type II. The result for both is the same—high blood sugar.

Would you put 20 teaspoons of sugar in your morning cup of coffee? That's precisely how much sugar the average American consumes daily. One can of soda alone contains a whopping nine teaspoons. High-sugar diets not only tax the pancreas, they can pack on the pounds, and 90 percent of type II diabetics are obese. Excess fat can keep cells from responding to insulin, so sugar stays in the blood. The longer it does, the higher your risk of heart disease, leg ulcers and even blindness. Julian Whitaker, author of *Reversing Diabetes*, points out that, "Ten years ago, type II diabetes was virtually unheard of in children. Today it is approaching epidemic proportions in children and adolescents." His explanation—25 percent of American children are overweight.

Sugar Consumption and Diabetes

An interesting study from Denmark shows the correlation between deaths due to diabetes and sugar consumption per one hundred thousand members of the population:

YEAR	DEATHS	SUGAR INTAKE PER PERSON/YEAR
1880	1.8	13.5 kg
1911	8.0	37.6 kg
1934	19.1	51.3 kg
1955	34.3	74.7 kg
1975	78.6	81.8 kg

The Diabetic Duo: One and Two

Insulin is required to absorb sugar from the blood into the body's cells, where it is used for energy. When insulin fails to be secreted from the pancreas (type I diabetes) sugar levels in the blood become very high and can cause serious health problems. There are two types of diabetes: type I diabetes and type II diabetes. Type I, also referred to as insulin-dependent diabetes, occurs when the pancreas stops producing enough insulin. Type I diabetes usually occurs before the age of twenty. Type II, or adult-onset diabetes, occurs when the body becomes less sensitive to the effects of insulin. In other words, there is plenty of insulin available but no way to use it. It is usually caused by the presence of too much body fat and can often be reduced or eliminated with weight loss, dietary changes and exercise. Type I diabetes is thought to be caused by an autoimmune disorder in which the immune system targets and destroys the cells of the pancreas that make insulin.

All Sugars Are Not Created Equal

Sugars to fight a blood sugar disease? While it may sound like an oxymoron, supplying the body with the right glyconutrients can help prevent and ease symptoms of diabetes. Glucose is public enemy number one in diabetes. Naturally, because glucose is formed from a number of dietary sugars (sucrose, fructose, galactose, etc.) the notion that there are sugars that could benefit the disease seems unlikely but is nevertheless true. For example, in type I diabetes, certain plant sugars may actually stimulate the pancreas to produce more insulin. Moreover, these sugars do so without causing the damaging side effects of high blood glucose levels. Glyconutrients cannot cure diabetes. They can, however, help to control its symptoms and minimize its complications.

Scientists at the Metabolic Research Laboratory in Minneapolis have found that mannose and galactose have the ability to increase insulin secretion. Another study published in the November 1997 issue of *Proceedings of the Fisher Institute for Medical Research* reported people with type I diabetes who were given dietary compounds that included mannose reported a dramatic improvement in their health, not to mention a decrease in vision problems, better wound healing, less infection, and lower blood pressure. In addition, some of the participants were able to lower their dosage of medicine.

Aloe Vera and Wound Healing in Diabetics

One of the terrible side effects of diabetes is slow wound healing, especially on the lower legs and feet. Several studies confirm that aloe vera inhibits inflammation and improves problematic wound healing in diabetics. The anti-inflammatory activity of aloe vera is well documented. The report suggests that a compound called gibberellin may be responsible for aloe vera's anti-inflammatory action. It also implies that compounds in aloe vera prompt wound healing through a different pathway than steroid drugs. Moreover, while steroids decrease inflammation, they also increase the risk of infection. By contrast, aloe vera inhibits inflammation but does not do so at the expense of healing.

Mannose and Diabetic Blindness

One of the worst complications of diabetes is the destruction of the retina by high levels of circulating blood sugar. The delicate retinal screen is literally "eaten away" by destructive proteins created by the presence of high blood sugar. In a study published in 1995, researchers at the Ophthalmology Department of Harvard University suggested that mannose might be able to substitute for glucose. Mannose has the ability to become the energy source for cells without the risk of eyesight damage. Of equal importance is that it could also work to stimulate the pancreas to produce more insulin, thereby lowering the amount of insulin needed to control this disease.

Medicinal Mushroom Sugars for Type I Diabetes

Type I diabetes occurs when the immune system mistakenly attacks the insulin-producing cells of the pancreas. Hence, even when a carbohydrate is consumed, insulin fails to enter the bloodstream. Several studies have emerged, and they suggest that fungi such as reishi or *Cordyceps sinensis* can prevent the development of type I diabetes in laboratory test animals predisposed to the disease. Moreover, cordyceps has also been tested in animals whose pancreas cells had been destroyed. The result: blood sugar was lowered, not by the action of insulin, but by the stimulation of a liver enzyme that metabolizes glucose. The bottom line is that both of these mushrooms were able to lower blood sugar through different pathways.

The "Glyco" Link to Complications of Diabetes

It's common for diabetics to also have a higher risk of cardiovascular disease. The simple explanation is that the presence of high blood sugar causes arteries to narrow. The more complex explanation deals with the type of glycoproteins found in people with diabetes. Researchers found that the glycoprotein content of platelets (the blood components involved in clotting) is usually impaired thereby increasing the risk of vascular events like stroke or heart attack. When sugar compounds stay in the blood, deranged proteins can be formed—proteins that can destroy retinal tissue in the eye and tiny blood vessels throughout the body.

Japanese scientists have recently discovered that the levels of a saccharide called N-acetylneuraminic acid-galactose (NANA-Gal) was abnormal in patients with complication of diabetes. The finding was so significant that they suggested that testing for NANA-Gal levels should be added to determine the health condition of a patient with diabetes. The innate relationship of sugars and sugar-bonded compounds in the human body and disease states is a profound one. In diabetes, it impacts virtually every body system and especially influences cardiovascular condition.

Hypoglycemia: Hype or Reality?

Technically speaking, hypoglycemia refers to low blood sugar (the opposite of diabetes), which occurs when levels drop too low to fuel physical activity. Medically speaking, hypoglycemia is rarely seen except as a side effect of receiving too much insulin, or from the presence of a tumor or hormone disorder. Now while I respect the technical definition of hypoglycemia, I can personally tell you that I do not have any of the above conditions, yet if I eat certain foods, my blood sugar drops low enough to spark a number of undesirable symptoms: shakiness, cold sweat, dizziness, weakness, intense hunger, and mental fogginess. In fact, after one encounter with a bowl of sugar frosted flakes, two hours later I became so weak I couldn't even stand up.

I soon discovered that when we eat foods high in simple carbohydrates, the pancreas overcompensates by secreting too much insulin, which inevitably brings our blood sugar levels down too low. Too much insulin can cause dramatic drops in blood sugar, which can result in shakiness, difficulty concentrating, cold sweats, fatigue, weakness and intense hunger. Hypoglycemia usually occurs one to three hours after eating a high-carbohydrate meal, such as refined cereals, pasta, bread or rice dishes. It is more likely to occur when these foods are eaten as a concentrated source of carbohydrates with little or no protein or fat. Diabetics can also experience hypoglycemia when insulin administration is poorly timed, if the person has exercised more than usual, or if the insulin dosage is too high.

The Perils of Low Blood Sugar

Normal blood sugar ranges in the 60 to 100 mg/dl of blood. When blood sugar drops below 50 mg/dl, the adrenal glands secrete adrenaline to prompt the release of stored sugar from the liver. This mechanism to compensate for low blood sugar is also associated with a number of symptoms that are individual specific and can include everything from short tempers to fainting. Interestingly, PMS is commonly accompanied by bouts with hypoglycemia, suggesting the hormonal impact of estrogen and progesterone on sugar and insulin mechanics. Individual biochemistry plays a role in whether an individual is prone to hypoglycemia and how severe their symptoms are. Naturally, diets high in carbohydrates can raise the risk of developing hypoglycemia. Symptoms of hypoglycemia include:

- hunger
- nervousness and shakiness
- perspiration
- dizziness or light-headedness
- sleepiness
- confusion
- difficulty in speaking
- feeling anxious or weak

Sugars That Keep Blood Sugar Levels "Level"

In a January issue of *Reproductive Nutrition and Development*, French researchers reported that the polysaccharides found in seaweed positively impacted blood sugar and insulin responses in laboratory animals. The addition of these polysaccharides resulted in what they described as a dramatically reduced glucose absorption balance. What this suggests is that polysaccharide compounds like fucoidan help to slow the infusion of glucose into the bloodstream from the intestines, thereby helping to keep blood sugar levels stable and prevent excessive insulin responses. For people with diabetes, insulin resistance or hypoglycemia, this is good news.

Beta-Glucans Benefit People with Blood Sugar Disorders

These remarkable sugars found in medicinal mushrooms and foods like oatmeal have a three-fold benefit for anyone who needs to control their blood sugar: they help to naturally lower blood sugar levels, they help control cholesterol and lipid levels in the blood, and they help prevent infection, which can be life threatening in diabetics.

Interestingly, a Swedish company has recently introduced a yogurt that is rich in beta-glucans to help maintain stable blood sugar and insulin levels in addition to lowering cholesterol. The yogurt contains 4 grams of beta-glucans derived from oats. Anyone suffering from diabetes should investigate supplements that contain beta-glucans. Aloe vera juice and fucoidan (found in brown seaweed products) are also important diabetes-related supplements.

Other Health Tips for Blood Sugar Problems

Increase Chromium Intake

Chromium tops the list by boosting insulin sensitivity so blood sugar levels are kept in check. People with type II diabetes were able to lower their medication with chromium supplementation. In 2002, a report published in *Diabetes Metabolism* recommended that we take a more serious look at chromium for diabetes prevention. Not surprisingly, low chromium levels correlate with an increased risk of type II diabetes.

Fats: Friends and Foes

Choose your fats wisely. Diabetes is linked to faulty fatty acid digestion. In the February 2001 issue of *Nutrition*, we read that fats rich in GLA (gamma-linolenic acid) protected animals against artificially induced diabetes. On the other hand, a study of eighty-five thousand women over fourteen years discovered that those consuming trans-fatty acids (compounds found in many margarines) significantly increased their risk of type II diabetes.

Mind Your Minerals

Studies show that ordinary zinc improves sugar metabolism by keeping insulin receptors sharp. And don't underestimate the role of magnesium. Almost one fourth of all people with type II diabetes lack magnesium. Vanadium, a trace mineral, actually mimics the effects of insulin, and in diabetic animals, it not only lowers blood sugar, but cholesterol levels as well. Adding vitamin E to the mineral mix is a good idea. Men with the lowest levels of vitamin E had nearly a four-times greater chance of developing type II diabetes.

Get Moving

"Every hour you spend in front of the TV increases your risk of type II diabetes," warns Dr. Julian Whitaker, well-known physician and author. He adds that, "Exercise increases insulin binding to various cells by 30 percent." In a study of 3,234 people who showed pre-diabetic symptoms, those who lost 5 to 7 percent of their body weight and moderately exercised for thirty minutes a day reduced their risk of getting type II diabetes by 58 percent.

Chapter Eight

Asthma, Allergies and Autoimmune Disease: Misguided Inflammation

"Disease is the retribution of outraged Nature." —*Hosea Ballou (1771-1852)*

Inflammation gone awry lies at the heart of asthma, allergies and autoimmune disease. These diseases result when an immune process designed to fight infection becomes the body's worst enemy. For example, when a pesky sliver gets under your skin, macrophages and other white blood cells rush to the site to fight the alien invader. As a result, the area becomes red, swollen and tender and stays that way until the rescue operation is complete, but sometimes the inflammatory response command is issued when it shouldn't be.

Asthma and most allergies deal with exaggerated or inappropriate inflammatory reactions. In asthma, irritation causes the bronchiole tubes in the lungs to constrict and eventually breakdown. Immune cells called neutrophils cause inflammation and are always present in bronchiole asthma attacks.

Allergies result from a similar phenomena, and autoimmune diseases occur from immune cells with the wrong mission statement—to sabotage its host (your body) by causing counterproductive inflammation in various locations. For example, in lupus, liver or kidney tissue can be targeted and subsequently becomes inflamed and even destroyed. For this reason, people with autoimmune diseases are typically placed on steroid drugs such as prednisone, which inhibits the inflammatory response.

Alleviating Allergies

Fifty million people suffer from assorted allergies, which include seasonal, chemical or food allergies. When trees and grasses pollinate, hay fever is the allergy "du jour." Pollen allergies cause itchy, watery eyes and runny noses. The pollen grains released by plants become airborne and settle in your nose. In allergy-prone people, a well-meaning but misguided immune system produces antibodies called immunoglobulin E (IgE) to fight pollen invaders. .

These antibodies stimulate an inflammatory response in the mast cells that line our nasal passages, eyes and skin. The result is a continual leak of histamine (sniff, sniff), the chemical responsible for sneezing, itching and congestion. The more mast cells you have, the more severe your allergic reaction. Interestingly, IgEs have also been implicated in food allergies. Certain foods like nuts, shellfish, wheat and milk can cause immediate or delayed allergic reactions that may include wheezing, coughing, bloating or diarrhea.

Routine medical treatment for pollen allergies involves antihistamines, mast cell blockers (cromolyn sodium) and corticosteroid nasal sprays. Over-the-counter nasal sprays, which shrink swollen membranes, can become habit-forming and if overused, can actually promote rebound congestion. Why some of us suffer with allergies and others don't still baffles doctors. Histamine is an inflammatory chemical released from mast cells during an allergic reaction. It's what irritates mucous membranes in the nose, eyes, throat and lungs.

Obviously, inhibiting histamine helps ease a whole host of miserable allergy symptoms.

The Histamine Blocker

Researchers belonging to the Faculty of Pharmaceutical Sciences at Kumamoto University, Japan, discovered that the sugar N-acetylneuraminic acid blocked the release of histamine (the culprit chemical in allergic reactions). Japanese researchers found that N-acetylneuraminic acid was able to decrease asthmatic bronchial spasms. In addition, L-fucose, a sugar found in brown seaweed and other sources, has been used to inhibit contact (allergic) dermatitis in test animals.

Incomplete digestion may cause tiny protein particles to trigger faulty immune reactions to pollen and specific foods. For this reason, some experts look at digestive enzyme supplementation as a first-line defense for allergies. "It is interesting to note that many inhalant allergies are eliminated when proper diet, improvement of digestion and enzyme therapy are employed," says Carolee Bateson-Koch in her book *Allergies: Diseases in Disguise*. Adding acidophilus (friendly bacteria) is also a good idea for food sensitivities. In one study, every child suffering from food allergies was deficient in friendly bowel bacteria (lactobacillus and bifidobacteria). In the old days, when humans ate plenty of fruits, plants, grains, seeds and nuts, the kind of intestinal flora residing in our colons was completely different. It contributed to rather than detracted from health.

Mannose Regulates Rogue Neutrophils

Mannose works to corral out-of-control neutrophils that cause misguided inflammation on a cellular level. Researchers at the Department of Microbiology and Immunology of the Hahnemann University School of Medicine confirmed that neutrophils (T cells) are suppressed by mannose. How? Scientists in Australia recently reported that immune T cells involved in the inflammatory response express mannose phosphate sugars on their surface. Consequently, they discovered that mannose phosphate controls the entry of T cells into inflammatory sites. In other words, mannose displaces certain enzymes required for T cells to flow into various places (joints, liver tissue, kidneys, etc.) thereby acting as a natural anti-inflammatory agent.

Controlling asthma, allergies and autoimmune disease boils down to normalizing misdirected immune reactions—something mannose appears to be capable of. Other studies confirm that it is a potent inhibitor of central nervous system inflammation. One such trial involved allergic encephalomyelitis, which scientists reported can be inhibited by various phosphosugars, but particularly by mannose-6-phosphate. They also concluded that mannose appears to negate the action of those enzymes that open the gates to immune inflammation activator cells.

Asthma

Asthma is a chronic condition that causes the constriction or narrowing, of the muscles surrounding the airways, combined with bronchiole inflammation and swelling. When airways become smaller, wheezing, coughing, chest tightness or shortness of breath can occur. In addition, continual irritation can cause the production of excess mucous, which only makes a bad situation worse.

An asthma attack can be absolutely terrifying, and if not controlled, can be fatal. Asthma is often triggered by allergies, infections, strong odors or fumes and exposure to cold or humid air. Like allergic reactions in the nose and eyes, the more asthma flares up, the more susceptible your lungs become to another attack. Once again, out-of-control inflammation is the culprit here and can exist even when obvious symptoms of asthma are absent. My mother suffered from severe asthma and used to rely on steroid drugs like prednisone to ease her inflamed bronchiole tubes. While steroid drugs do block the inflammatory response, they come with potentially serious side effects.

Glyconutrients to Ease Asthma

Because glyconutrients help to calm inflammation and restore immune balance, taking them for an inflammatory condition like asthma makes perfect sense—a notion based on the fact that when therapeutic sugars are present in the right amounts, an overstimulated immune system can be tamed on an enzymatic level. Unfortunately, at this writing no long-term, double-blind studies exist that scientifically support the beneficial use of glyconutrients for asthma. There have been, however, several anecdotal studies suggesting that taking a complete array of glyconutrients inhibits the lung inflammation associated with asthma and does so safely and without side effects of steroid or other drugs. A new study confirms that a correlation exists between lung function and patterns of inflammation. A study published in the *American Journal of Respiratory Critical Care Medicine* in 2000 reported that a glycoprotein (alpha-1-acid glycoprotein) contains several sugar molecules whose branching patterns relate to immune activity. In other words, abnormal branching in this glycoprotein aggravates lung inflammation—a finding that suggests people with asthma have deranged or abnormal glycoprotein configurations.

Fucoidan (found in brown seaweed) is another polysaccharide that caused a 96.8 percent reduction in neutrophil invasion (the vehicles of inflammation) even at a relatively small dose. Remember that neutrophils are recruited into inflammatory sites by the adhesion of immune messenger cells to other cells. Apparently, fucoidan helps to stop this from occurring. There is also some preliminary evidence that consuming the "essential eight" sugars together may also help ease the symptoms of chronic asthma.

Note: Like other serious diseases, no one should discontinue their medications in exchange for any supplementation without the approval and supervision of their physician.

Mannose-Binding Lectin: Are You Deficient?

Mannose-binding lectin (MBL) is an incredible and highly versatile immune macro-molecule. In the presence of calcium this amazing protein can bind to a wide spectrum of sugar arrays. This "binding" ability makes it possible for a phagocyte (immune germ-eater) to attach to a microbial surface where it can do its job. Of particular interest—experts have recently discovered that low levels of MBL or mutated MBL may indicate compromised immunity. A correlation was found between an increased incidence of infections in individuals low in MBL. In other words, the phenomena was commonly found in people with immune deficiencies, frequent unexplained infections, and those with systemic lupus erythematosus. There is also evidence that abnormal MBL causes AIDS in HIV-positive men to progress faster. Interestingly, even children who are prone to infections are significantly more likely to be lacking in normal MBL proteins. Moreover, inadequate MBL was also associated with early manifestation of autoimmune disease in immune-compromised individuals. In fact, the mean age of disease onset was 14.5 years in people with low producing MBL

A New Way to Screen for Immune Deficiency

A recent study published in the *Annals of Allergy, Asthma & Immunology* involved taking blood samples from the blood bank of the Mayo Clinic. They represented a population of blood donors living in the Midwest. They randomly selected 148 samples from both men and women. They found that a mannose-binding lectin deficiency plays a dramatic role in the development of primary immune deficiency in humans. They suggest physicians should screen patients with recurrent infections and autoimmune disease for a lack of mannose-binding lectin.

To my way of thinking, supplying the immune system of both children and adults with dietary mannose would be the first step in addressing this immune protein malfunction. It's not a stretch to assume that a dietary deficiency of glyconutrients like mannose could ostensibly contribute to a MBL-related problem. Scientists do know that the oral consumption of mannose elevates blood mannose levels. In fact, they refer to this rudimentary action as the first step toward an effective therapy for people who are glycoprotein deficient.

The Anti-Allergy Duo

Good ol' vitamin C helps to detoxify cells of histamine. One study found that the histamine level of every person given one gram of vitamin C daily for three days declined. Remember that the less histamine, the less inflammation.

The addition of quercetin (a bioflavonoid) potentiates the anti-allergy actions of vitamin C by inhibiting the release of histamine from mast cells in people with hay fever. You don't want to take one without the other.

Other Sources of Allergy Relief

- *Xylitol:* Using a nasal wash preparation that contains xylitol, (a natural sugar) can help keep some bacteria from sticking to cells so post-allergy infection is less likely to occur. Unlike over-the-counter nasal sprays, xylitol varieties are safe and non-habit forming.
- *Digestive Enzymes:* Look for full-strength products with pancreatin.
- *Probiotics (Lactobacillus Acidophilus):* Use nondairy products with guaranteed bacterial count as directed. Keep refrigerated.
- *Vitamin C with Bioflavonoids (Especially Quercetin):* Use buffered forms for less stomach upset.
- *Change Your Home Environment:* Consider installing an air purifier and change your bed sheets/pillow cases often.

Autoimmune Diseases and Glyconutrients

When immune cells mistake the good guys for the bad guys and engage in cell-to-cell combat, autoimmune diseases can develop. In fostering autoimmune disease, the immune system basically cuts off its nose to spite its face. Why? Because it has received corrupted data and carries out self-destructive orders. The mechanisms of the immune system protect us against harmful antigens that include microorganisms, toxins, cancer cells, and foreign blood or tissues. Immune cells see and destroy antigens by using antibodies that adhere to an antigen marking it for destruction and by sending specialized white blood cells to destroy it.

An autoimmune disease develops when the immune system destroys normal body tissues. In other words, the system goes into overdrive and reacts to the presence of normal cells it should normally leave alone. It becomes unable to tell the difference between the enemy and itself, so the body becomes a casualty of "friendly fire." Immune lymphocytes override their normal suppression by other lymphocytes not to attack body tissues. Simply stated, normal controls fail and cellular codes give out faulty instructions causing inflammation and subsequent tissue destruction.

Consequently red blood cells, connective tissues, and endocrine glands such as the thyroid or pancreas, the liver, kidneys, muscles, joints and skin can all be targeted. As a result, symptoms can vary. Why this destructive phenomena occurs remains unknown. Everything from hidden viruses to stress to vaccinations have been implicated in autoimmune disorders. The one thing they all have in common is displaced inflammation.

Examples of Faulty Immune Data Transmissions

- *Multiple Sclerosis:* Immune cells are misinstructed to attack the myelin sheathes that cover our nerves.
- *Lupus:* Immune cells mistakenly attack the liver or skin.
- *Psoriasis:* Certain skin cells don't get the "quittin' time" message and continue to grow into thick plaques.
- *Type I Diabetes:* Immune cells are misinstructed to attack islet cells in the pancreas that make insulin.
- *Rheumatoid Arthritis:* Immune cells are misinstructed to attack cartilage cushions in joints.
- *Crohn's Disease:* Immune cells are misinstructed to attack bowel tissue.

As you can see from this varied list, immune attack cells can mistakenly destroy tissue located anywhere in the body. Known autoimmune disorders include:

- Hashimoto's thyroiditis
- pernicious anemia
- Addison's disease
- diabetes
- rheumatoid arthritis
- systemic lupus erythematosus
- dermatomyositis
- Sjogren's syndrome
- multiple sclerosis
- myasthenia gravis
- Reiter's syndrome
- Graves disease

Conventional Treatment for Autoimmune Diseases

Ideally, a natural treatment would be able to reduce symptoms and suppress immune attack cells without compromising resistance to disease. Corticosteroids to block inflammation and immuno-suppressant medications like cyclophosphamide or azathioprine may be prescribed but come with significant side effects. Unfortunately medical science can only offer victims of autoimmune diseases symptomatic relief. To date, a cure has not been found. What needs to be emphasized here is that when immune cells attack healthy tissue, a massive breakdown in cell-to-cell communications has occurred—a process that depends on the function of healthy glycoforms or sugar molecules.

Fighting Arthritis with Glyconutrients

In rheumatoid arthritis, the process of inflammation goes into overdrive and cartilage that normally cushions and lubricates our joints is destroyed by our own immune cells. While osteoarthritis is considered a result of "wear and tear," rheumatoid arthritis is considered an autoimmune disease. Although hidden viruses and bacteria have been suspected as the real cause of rheumatoid arthritis, the jury is still out. The deranged immune response to a glycoprotein that is found in human cartilage is responsible for the inflammation that causes rheumatoid arthritis.

Not surprisingly, studies suggest that L-fucose (fucoidan) is low in people with rheumatoid arthritis, and its supplementation is described as a promising treatment since it is "a safe and simple natural sugar." What is particularly interesting is that the lower a person's level of fucose is, the more advanced their rheumatoid arthritis.

Moreover, according to the work of Doris Lefkowitz, Ph.D., the severity of rheumatoid arthritis has also been linked to low galactose levels and vice-versa. According to her report, the vicious cycle of inflammation seen in arthritis is caused by abnormal "cross-talk" between immune cells.

Mannose is also crucial for joint protection. When laboratory test animals received mannans (polymers of mannose), inflammation flare ups were prevented. And like other diseases we've discussed, genetic mutations in, or a lack of, mannose-binding proteins can predispose a person to rheumatoid arthritis. Providing the body with glyconutrients appears to correct the miscommunication between immune cells that causes autoimmune diseases like rheumatoid arthritis. Two other sugars (N-acetylglucosamine and N-acetylgalactosamine) also work in the joints to sweep up destructive free radicals in joints that form during any inflammation. These sugars also keep well-intentioned but misguided immune attack cells from sticking to healthy cells.

While it may come as a surprise to many, some forms of arthritis appear to occur after bouts with intestinal infections. In addition, Dutch scientists recently reported that chronic arthritis may have a bacterial connection. In fact, if you suffer from rheumatoid arthritis, which is considered an autoimmune disease, your disease may have been triggered by a prior infection that may have overstimulated immune responses that, in this scenario, need suppressing.

N-Acetylglucosamine: Joint-Friendly Sugar

If you suffer from osteoarthritis, which is not considered an autoimmune disease, and take NSAIDs (non-steroidal anti-inflammatory drugs) for pain and swelling, the natural anti-inflammatory effect of glyconutrients can also be of great benefit. Glucosamine has already gained celebrity status for its ability to stimulate the regeneration of cartilage in damaged joints and has been the subject of countless studies. It does indeed prompt healing, reduce swelling and increase flexibility. Of equal importance, joint injuries may heal more rapidly if the body is supplemented with N-acetylglucosamine. One study suggests that its addition actually reduced cartilage damage following a knee injury.

Multiple Sclerosis: An Overview

Multiple sclerosis (MS) is another autoimmune disease in which the immune system targets the myelin sheathes that provide a protective covering for nerve cells. Symptoms of the disease can vary depending on the location of the nerve cell attack. MS afflicts one in seven hundred people in this country and currently there is no cure for the disease. While several studies suggest that abnormal fatty acid metabolism may be involved in MS, medical practitioners remain generally unaware that a lack of certain glyconutrients is linked to the disease.

MS: A Sugar-Deficient Disease?

What is not commonly known is that MS has been linked to the inability to absorb xylose and to the presence of abnormal galactose molecules. Interestingly, the myelin sheath that covers our nerves and is attacked by immune cells in MS contains galactose. This being the case, galactose and xylose supplementation may have a corrective effect. Furthermore, because acemannan (derived from aloe) has several beneficial effects on the immune system, its use for people with MS is scientifically supported. Studies have found that acemannan modulates the immune system, enhances cell regeneration, and fights viral infection.

Could MS Be Linked to Infection?

A startling report was found in the July 1999 issue of *Annals of Neurology*. Researchers reported that a common bacterium called *Chlamydia pneumoniae* was present in all the patients tested in the study with multiple sclerosis. This bacteria is the same one that causes walking pneumonia. While MS has been classified as an autoimmune disorder in which the immune system's defense mechanisms mistakenly destroy the nerve coverings, new studies tell us that a bacteria may really be to blame.

A viral link has also been discovered to MS. Recent data from the Institute of Neurological Disorders and Stroke indicated the presence of a herpes virus in 30 percent of people tested with MS. In both of these scenarios, it is thought that the infectious agent remains dormant in nerve tissue until a flair up. If MS involves both an overactive and underactive immune system, finding a treatment that can address both needs simultaneously evades modern medicine. Not surprisingly, Mother Nature has already beaten medical science to the punch. Sugars like mannose are able to control both underactive and overactive immune systems.

Inflammatory Bowel Diseases

Inflammatory bowel disease refers to Crohn's disease and ulcerative colitis in which the immune system attacks tissue in the intestine. Subsequent symptoms may include diarrhea, nausea, vomiting, abdominal cramps and pain. Once again, the inflammatory response is at fault and once again prescribing high doses of corticosteroid (prednisone) therapy is used to control severe symptoms—a practice that can predispose patients to infections, bone thinning and fractures. More than one in five hundred Americans has some type of inflammatory bowel disease. Studies conclusively show that a test group of people with colitis have problems with the monosaccharide (sugar) function in their colons. Even more telling is that over half of the healthy subjects in one study published in *Clinical Science* contained all eight essential sugars in the mucus lining of the bowel as compared to barely a fourth of the people with bowel disease. Acemannan has also been recommended to check the inflammation associated with a variety of bowel disorders.

Systemic Lupus Erythematosus

Lupus is another in a long list of poorly understood autoimmune diseases. Lupus affects thousands of people each year, yet we still know little about the disease. It is characterized by chronic inflammation that can affect various parts of the body, especially the skin, joints, blood and kidneys. If you have lupus, your immune system makes antibodies that are against yourself hence the term *auto-antibodies*. These entities react with antigens found on healthy tissue to form abnormal immune complexes and build up in the tissues causing inflammation and tissue destruction. The extent to which this happens differentiates a mild disease that periodically targets a few organs from a serious and potentially life-threatening one. More than sixteen thousand Americans develop lupus each year and up to 1.5 million Americans have been diagnosed with lupus.

Dysfunctional Mannose Bonds and Lupus

Lupus has also been linked to abnormalities and deficiencies of mannose-binding proteins. The same thing was found in people with dermatomyositis, which is also discussed in this chapter. In 1996, the Sullivan study published in *Arthritis and Rheumatism* concluded that a low level of mannose-binding proteins may make a person susceptible to lupus.

One recent study concluded that the presence of dysfunctional mannose-binding proteins in a group of Spanish test subjects was a significant risk factor for developing lupus. The same results were obtained in another study of a group of Japanese patients with lupus.

Dermatomyositis

Dermatomyositis (a disease of connective tissue with arthritis-like symptoms) is characterized by sugars whose structures changed after a parasitic infection. We've already established that whenever the "glyco" or sugar part of a molecule is altered, communication channels between immune agents can break down and the wrong commands can be given. This is one of several autoimmune diseases that show the same profile: a lack of dietary sugars, the inability to absorb them, or abnormalities in their structures. As mentioned earlier, a new study disclosed that once again a lack of mannose-binding proteins is associated with dermatomyositis.

Can Autoimmune Diseases Be Prevented?

Research tells us that glyconutrient supplementation may actually prevent autoimmune diseases. Several studies suggest that a dietary deficiency of certain sugars may spark the development of autoimmune diseases. In fact, the Newkirk study published in a 1996 issue of *Clinical and Experimental Immunology* (and others) found that galactose deficiencies were common in almost all cases of autoimmune disease. Moreover, scientists at the Department of Cellular and Molecular in London confirmed that abnormal cellular sugar structures can cause antibodies to attack healthy tissue. Remember that cellular messages direct the show. In other words, if the "glycogram" telegraphs the wrong message, immune attack cells will turn on the body. Glycomolecules actually tell immune cells when and where to mount an attack.

Human tissue that is continually attacked by misinformed immune cells is subject to chronic inflammation that causes pain and cell destruction leading to prolonged illness or even death. While conventional medications (prednisone, methotrexate, cyclophosphamide, azathioprine, and cyclosporin) help to manage symptoms of autoimmune diseases, they also suppress the body's ability to fight infection and have other potentially serious side effects. Normalizing inappropriate immune pathways of inflammation with few side effects would be the best-case scenario. The use of therapeutic sugars for anyone with an autoimmune disease should be investigated for its powerful anti-inflammatory effect.

Chapter Nine

The Glyconutrient-Cancer Connection

"Nobody knows what the cause is, though some pretend they do;
it is like some hidden assassin waiting to strike at you. Childless
women get it, and men when they retire; it is as if there had to be
some outlet for their foiled creative fire." –*W. H. Auden*

One in every three Americans will develop cancer. Approximately 1.2 million cancer cases are diagnosed every year in this country, and that number is going up—not down, despite all of the research and attention devoted to it. Of these cases, six in ten people will die within five years. Cancer is a worldwide scourge that continues to elude a cure. Its causes are diverse, but its mission is always the same—to snuff out life. You can develop cancer in virtually any part of your body, including your blood and bones.

In my view, cancer could appropriately be called an immune-deficiency disease. It exemplifies a serious breach of immune function. The million-dollar question is why cancer is allowed to grow in certain people and not in others—moreover, can a person with cancer change its course by waking up the very immune cells that have failed them?

Stated simply, cancer is characterized by the uncontrolled growth of abnormal cells that are permitted to reproduce due to a serious immune collapse. In essence, cancer is allowed to grow unchecked because our immune surveillance system falls asleep. John Bailar, M.D., Ph.D., former editor-in-chief of the *Journal of the National Cancer Institute* said, "For cancer to start and then continue growing, it must outmaneuver the many long arms of your immune defenses. The immune system is both your first and last defense against cancer."

Immune watch-guard cells normally identify and destroy cancer cells. Immune cells called B-lymphocytes produce antibodies specifically designed to destroy malignant cells. What baffles experts is why the system breaks down so the presence of cancer cells fails to trigger normal alarm mechanisms in some people.

How Does Cancer Fool the Immune System?

Cancer cells fly below the immune system's radar screen so their presence remains undetected by the very defenders that should "seek and destroy" them. Recently, scientists at Stanford University set up a method to measure immune function as it relates to cancer development. Apparently their findings support the notion that people who get cancer have plenty of immune watch-dog cells present, but they fail to spring into action—seemingly desensitized to the presence of the enemy, so they do nothing. Some experts believe this "incapacitation" is actually triggered by the presence of cancer cells, which in some cases put the warning system to sleep. So why do some immune defenders attack a cancer cell why others do not?

If a cancer cell produces an antigen signature, a red flag goes up and the immune system is alerted to the presence of an intruder. Pathologists routinely find anticancer immune cells in tumors or lymph nodes—a fact that indicates that immune defenders were vigilant. Regardless of this recognition, cancer will often still grow and even spread. Obviously, the development of cancer goes beyond a simple recognition failure. One fascinating study isolated these anticancer cells for the sole purpose of testing their responsiveness. Through an extraordinary technique, they were able to identify, count and isolate killer T cells from blood samples of people with melanoma that had already metastasized or spread. In almost half the samples, they detected the presence of a significant number of killer T cells that were attacking the melanoma. It appeared as though the immune system was aggressively going after the cancer, but the presence of the advanced cancer said otherwise.

Further investigation revealed that the killer T cells did not respond as they should. For instance, when a sample of the T cells were put in contact with melanoma cells, nothing happened. The protein they should have produced in the process of the attack was missing. The cancer antigens failed to evoke the proper response. Interestingly this lack of action was seen only in the T cells that reacted to cancer cells. Other types had the proper reaction to viruses. The inevitable conclusion is the presence of cancer may signal inhibited killer T cell activity against cancer antigens. The likely reason: cancer cells preserve themselves by disabling immune defenders. If you have cancer, it means that their strategy has succeeded.

Stated simply, if you have faulty immune responses, you are at a much higher risk of developing cancer. None of us can completely avoid our exposure to pollution, pesticides, additives and ultra-violet rays. It is crucial to arm natural immune defenders with all the raw materials they need to protect the human body against cancer and other diseases.

When a Fail-Safe System Fails

Why is a rogue cancer cell permitted to grow in some people? Cancer is a clever disease that fools even the best built-in safeguards of the immune system. New evidence suggests that cancerous cells dodge detection by the immune system in one of two ways. Immunology and cancer researchers found that a protective immune protein called interferon-gamma is incapacitated when cancer is allowed to grow. In other words, its early warning system becomes inactivated. This phenomena may explain why giving some patients interferon did nothing to slow tumor growth. The role of interferon is what triggers other immune responses. The ability of a cancer cell to paralyze the immune system appears to depend on genetic factors and on the type of cancer cell present.

How Plant-Rich Diets Fight Cancer

We all know that our diets are profoundly linked to the formation of cancer, and yet most of us continue to eat poorly. One reason a diet rich in fresh fruits and vegetables is cancer preventive is due to its glyconutrient and other phytochemical content. The general consensus among scores of health experts is that our current obsession with high-protein, high-fat, highly refined foods puts our immune systems at an increased risk for phytonutrient depletion. When was the last time you saw a kid eating an orange?

Unquestionably, a reduced cancer risk is associated with diets high in plant foods. Vegetables, fruits, seeds and nuts contain live enzymes, scores of cancer-protective biochemicals and fiber, which has a long list of health benefits.

Glycoproteins and Cancer

Unquestionably, the abnormal formation of glycoproteins in the immune arena plays a significant role in the development of cancer. In fact, some scientists believe that mutated or dysfunctional glycoproteins are predictors of cancer formation. As we already talked about, almost all key players in the immune system rely on glycoproteins to accomplish their mission. One report in the August, 1996 *Journal of Pathology* stated, "Tumor development is usually associated with changes in cell surface carbohydrates."

Abnormal mannose and N-acetylglucosamine sugars have been found in breast and colon cancer cells. In addition, a lack of monosaccharide sugars have been linked to the spread of cancer cells throughout the body. Similarly, cancer of the gastrointestinal tract may result from a lack of monosaccharide consumption. Experts tell us that when a glycoprotein is altered, it can impact how cancer cells attach to healthy cells and how they reproduce and spread. Of even more importance, malfunctioning glycoproteins may cause immune T cells to become incapacitated after they encounter cancer cells. Glyconutrients with proven antitumor properties include mannose, glucose, galactose, glucosamine, fucose and polysaccharide K.

Mannose and Cancer-Eating Cells

Proteins that carry mannose sugars on their surface can actually stimulate macrophages to literally "devour" cancer cells. Moreover, when mannose binds to these cells, it activates macrophage action and also initiates the secretion of other substances (like interferon), which alert and reinforce other immune defenses. By so doing, the growth of cancerous tumors is inhibited.

Glyconutrients and Cancer: The Track Record

Glyconutrients should be used as part of a complete cancer-fighting protocol that includes diet, conventional medicine and stress management. In my mind, there is no doubt that these plant sugars provide extremely valuable support in boosting natural immune functions that fight cancer. Moreover, these sugars can enhance the efficacy of conventional treatments and boost infection resistance. Here are a few bits of data that support the benefits of glyconutrients for people with cancer.

- Arabinogalactan, which has a galactose backbone, can stimulate the immune system enough to block the spread of liver cancer cells.
- Injections of fucose in laboratory test animals have shown promise as a breast cancer treatment.
- U-fucoidan, a complex polysaccharide found in brown seaweed, was able to kill cancer cells in vitro within seventy-two hours. Interestingly the destruction was self-induced. The sugars were able to break down the DNA within each cancer cell through the action of enzymes. This process of self-destruction is known as "apoptosis."
- When scientists added sugars including D-mannose, D-ribose, and D-glucosamine into the drinking water of mice with tumor cells, their survival rate was increased and tumor rate decreased.
- Xylose supplementation may prevent cancers of the digestive system.
- Some studies concluded that fucose and mannose appeared to be the most effective sugars when it came to slowing the growth of cancer cells.
- Lentinan, found in shiitake mushrooms, has marked anti-tumor activity and prevents cancer recurrence or spread after surgery. In addition, it also helps mitigate the side effects of chemotherapy.
- Polysaccharide K (PSK), also known as krestin and found in a fungus called *Coriolus versicolor*, is a protein-bound

polysaccharide that has been used as a chemo-immunotherapy agent in the treatment of cancer in Asia for decades. Several clinical trials have shown that PSK has enormous potential as an adjuvant cancer therapy agent. Beneficial results have been reported in cases of stomach, esophageal, colorectal, breast and lung cancers. Apparently, PSK enhances the "host versus tumor response," thereby boosting the ability of the immune system to fight tumor progression and has important antioxidant actions as well.

Four Ways Glyconutrients Fight Cancer

First, they stimulate macrophage and immune killer cells to destroy cancer (first line of defense). Then, they increase the production of substances like interferon to target and destroy malignant cells. They also activate T cells to recognize invaders and destroy them (second line of defense). Finally, they assist in determining when cells die off (apoptosis). If this safety mechanism fails, cancer cells are allowed to keep replicating.

No one should start on any glyconutrient supplementation without consulting their physician. And large doses should be divided into increments of 500 mg.

Glyconutrients for Chemotherapy Support

Chemotherapy involves administering certain drugs to treat cancer and other diseases. Its upside? It can kill cancer cells found throughout the body. Its downside is that it is also toxic to healthy cells found throughout the body. More than one hundred different drugs are used in various combinations for individual cases of cancer. Common side effects of chemotherapy include fatigue, nausea, pain, hair loss and ane-

mia. Moreover, people on chemotherapy can become susceptible to all kinds of infections because chemo weakens the
immune system. It does so because anticancer drugs impact
rapidly dividing cells in the immune system and elsewhere.
That's why people receiving chemo typically lose their hair.

There are two primary reasons why supplementation with
glyconutrients can benefit anyone undergoing chemotherapy.
First, some sugars actually work to potentiate the actions of
chemotherapy on cancer cells. Second, providing therapeutic
sugars to the immune system during chemotherapy helps prevent vulnerability to infections and other unwanted side
effects.

For example, one study found in a 1994 issue of *Lancet*
found that a group of patients with stomach cancer who took
polysaccharide K in combination with chemotherapy had a
higher five-year survival rate than those who were treated
with chemotherapy alone. Treatment with lentinan (contained
in shiitake mushrooms) also helps ease the side effects associated with chemotherapy while enhancing resistance against
infections from various types of bacteria, viruses, fungi and
parasites with no toxicity.

Glyconutrients for Chemotherapy and Radiation Treatments

- mannose (aloe vera)
- lentinan (shiitake mushrooms)
- fucose (fucoidan, from brown seaweed)
- polysaccharides K and P (various mushrooms, *Coriolus versicolor, Cordyceps sinensis*)
- beta-glucans family
- maitake D-fraction (maitake mushroom)

Other Supplements That Fight Cancer

Astragalus

This herb, also known in Chinese medicine as huang chi, may help fight cancer by stimulating defense cells in the immune system. Researchers have found that when astragalus was mixed with the blood of cancer patients in vitro, the action of cancer-killing T lymphocyte cells improved by 260 percent.

Borage Oil (GLA)

Borage oil contains a compound called gamma linolenic acid (GLA), which has the ability to kill brain and prostate cancer cells and to slow the spread of malignant tumors by inhibiting the growth of blood vessels that nourish the tumor.

Indole-3-Carbinol

Indole-3-carbinol is an anticancer substance found in cruciferous (cabbage family) vegetables and belongs to a class of sulfur-containing chemicals called glucosinolates.

Transfer Factors

Isolated from cow colostrum, transfer factors empower immune response by adding immune data that stimulates better immune function. Asian studies reveal that TF can also keep the immune system strong during chemotherapy. Studies also reveal that using transfer factors may improve the chances of a cancer-free future.

Calcium D-Glucarate (D-Glucaric Acid)

Studies show taking D-glucarate orally prompts a slow release of a substance that inhibits an enzyme that prevents the immune system from neutralizing cancer-causing substances. Seventy percent of rats given a chemical that induces breast cancer that were pre-treated with dietary glucarate did not develop tumors. The trial also discovered that glucarate lowered blood levels of estradiol (the form of estrogen that causes breast cancer).

Coenzyme Q10 (CoQ10)

Studies of women with breast cancer suggest that CoQ10 supplements combined with conventional treatments may help to shrink tumors and contribute to partial remission in some women.

Chapter Ten

Heart Disease:
An Inflammatory Condition?

"A man's health can be judged by which he takes two
at a time—pills or stairs." *–Joan Welsh*

For years doctors have told us that the primary cause of heart disease is high cholesterol, which comes from eating too many saturated fats and living a sedentary lifestyle. When the situation reaches the crisis stage, the medical solution has been to snip out the offending sections of a clogged artery (bypass surgery) and send the patient on their way. There is a growing body of evidence, however, indicating that instead of reaming or replacing our "pipes" to deal with cholesterol deposits, we should be adding certain nutrients to the liquid that flows through them. New studies show that inflammatory responses that impact artery walls make them much more likely to collect cholesterol and become blocked.

Inflammation: The Hidden Killer

A recent study reveals that heart failure is similar to other chronic illnesses in which a low-grade chronic inflammatory process is at work. In other words, the immune inflammatory process causes continual tissue wasting in the heart muscle. Cytokines from the immune system are the culprits and cell-to-cell chatter gone wrong is at the heart of the phenomena. Consider this quote from the same study, "Although the inciting event is located in the heart, cross-talk between the myocardium on the one hand, and the immune system, peripheral tissues and organs on the other hand, will lead to the overproduction of proinflammatory cytokines and, inevitably, to their detrimental effects."

Likewise, researchers have also found that regardless of dietary and lifestyle changes and the use of cholesterol-lowering drugs, coronary heart disease remains the major cause of death in this country. Consequently, experts have concluded that coronary artery disease is not simply the result of arterial plaque accumulations but is caused by an on-going inflammatory process activated by faulty cellular interactions.

Targeting Inflammatory Cytokines

Doctors have been slow to acknowledge, detect and treat the immune inflammatory link to heart disease, which if screened for, could prevent countless heart operations. More importantly, understanding how inflammation impacts heart disease is just beginning to emerge. Inflammatory components can irritate blood vessel walls causing them to accumulate plaque and narrow. Much like rubbing sandpaper on a nylon stocking, inflammation causes snags to develop in artery walls. These "snags" attract lipids and they collect and grow around them. Interestingly, some studies suggest that the use of anti-inflammatory drugs can prevent heart attacks and strokes. Unfortunately, the long-term use of aspirin and NSAIDs (non-steroidal anti-inflammatory drugs) can create serious gastrointestinal side effects.

Beware of Over-the Counter Pain Killers for Colds and Flu

Most of us are quick to grab aspirin or ibuprofen when we are beset with the unpleasant symptoms that accompany colds and flu. Ironically, these medicines may actually prolong the duration of these infections by suppressing immune function. Clinical trials found that when subjects with colds used these medications, they experienced a decreased production of antibodies and a worsening of nasal symptoms. The old fashioned belief that suppressing symptoms may actually prolong them emerges as a distinct possibility here. One of the primary differences between conventional and holistic medicine is the notion that symptomatic relief alone may not only impede healing, but it also neglects to target the root cause of disease. Artificially lowering a fever with aspirin or other drugs may actually be counterproductive in some instances. If a fever doesn't get too high, it can actually boost immune function to more quickly kill infectious organisms. So, before you reach for that bottle, you may want to consider letting nature take its course.

C-Reactive Protein: Predictor of Heart Attacks

Recently a landmark study came up with a conclusion that has doctors reeling—it turns out that your level of something called C-reactive protein (CRP) may be the single most reliable predictor of your risk of heart attack or stroke. C-reactive protein is released by the body in response to an injury, infection or inflammation. Because plaque that is stuck to artery walls typically contains inflammatory cells, your level of CRP can act as an indicator of plaque deposits and atherosclerosis. CRP levels confirm the presence of arterial inflammation.

Studies confirm that a positive link between CRP and coronary artery disease exists. In a survey of 388 British men aged fifty to sixty-nine, the prevalence of coronary artery disease increased 1.5 fold for each doubling of CRP level. Elevated CRP levels indicate the presence of inflammation that can cause heart disease and subsequent heart attack and strokes. Conservatively speaking, it is thought that almost one fourth the population has elevated CRP levels, making their risk of a heart attack significantly higher, even if their cholesterol levels are normal, giving them a false sense of security. It's frightening to think that many of us harbor this inflammatory threat to our heart without knowing it.

Bugs in the Arteries

Another way to find out if you're a candidate for heart disease is to check your levels of interleukin-1, an inflammatory marker of an underlying infection. A new article published in the *New England Journal of Medicine* found that up to 55 percent of heart attacks appear to be prevented by treatment with proper antibiotics. Moreover, evidence published in the February 1999 issue of *Science* points to an infectious bacteria known as chlamydia. In addition, cytomegalo virus and herpes have also been closely linked to heart attacks. Chlamydia is abundant in our environment, and most of us have probably been exposed to the infection, which is thought to enter the body and lodge in arterial plaque. Most of us are routinely exposed to these microorganisms that, in some cases, negatively impact the lining of our arteries. These studies imply that the inability of the immune system to eradicate these invaders may lie at the real "heart" of heart disease. The question is, Why does this happen in some people? Could sugar molecules that lack their protein "spouse" be to blame?

Heart Disease and Sugarless Proteins

Scientists have discovered that groups of people who were heart attack survivors had a much higher count of proteins that were without attached sugars. These "headless" proteins were often missing their glucosamine sugar mates. Interestingly, researchers at the National Institute of Food and Nutrition in Warsaw discovered that their "sugarless" state correlated to higher cholesterol and blood fat levels.

Russian scientists found that healthy people with good LDL cholesterol levels have a certain ratio of N-acetylglycosamine, galactose, mannose and N-acetylneuramine in their blood. What does this all mean? It tells us that keeping heart muscle continually supplied with glyconutrients is vital to its protection and repair. It even suggests that a lack or malfunction of these sugars and proteins may initiate the beginnings of heart disease—the collection of cholesterol on artery walls.

Mannose and Heart Disease

A recent study has found that a disease that involves the inflammation of coronary blood vessels in children is linked to mannose-binding lectin. The study emphasizes that young children primarily rely on their innate immune system for protection against invading microorganisms, of which mannose-binding lectin is a vital component. The study looked at ninety patients who had a higher frequency of mutations in the MBL gene than healthy children. They found that children younger than one year with the mutations were at higher risk of development of coronary artery lesions. They concluded that the innate immune system contributes to the pathophysiology of this coronary vessel condition. Findings like this and others further support the idea that mannose plays a profound role in proper immune response.

Using Glyconutrients to Fight Coronary Inflammation

Like any other disorder, a successful treatment strategy for heart health must involve dietary and lifestyle changes coupled with supplementation. The inflammatory link to heart disease, however, suggests that targeting the cells that cause inflammation with certain compounds may be extremely important to heart health. The following nutrients contain saccharides that boost heart health by fighting hidden infections and inflammation and lower cholesterol levels as well:

- aloe vera
- psyllium
- *Cordyceps sinensis*
- beta-glucans
- fucose

Using Mannose for Heart Health

Mannose supplementation (found in aloe vera) offers several benefits for heart health. Mannose has natural and powerful anti-inflammatory actions; it works to suppress or enhance immune function as needed; and if you have markers of inflammation, it can modulate the inflammatory response. Moreover, if a hidden infection is to blame, mannose works to rev up the action of killer T cells for better immune response to foreign invaders.

Glyconutrients That Lower Bad Cholesterol

I used to think that eating oatmeal lowered cholesterol levels because of its high fiber content. While that assumption is technically true, I was surprised to learn that oats contain the glyconutrient family of beta-glucans. These sugars that are also found in medicinal mushrooms are contained in both oatmeal and barley grain and have proven abilities to reduce blood cholesterol concentrations. In fact, consuming these cereals works to lower the risk of stroke or heart attack, to lower cholesterol, and to promote intestinal health.

Studies tell us that 3 grams or more daily of beta-glucan soluble fiber from whole oats, as part of a diet low in saturated fat and cholesterol, may reduce the risk of heart disease. Beta-glucans are also found in baker's yeast. The U.S. Food and Drug Administration (FDA) has approved beta-glucan to reduce cardiovascular disease risk.

Consuming psyllium can also reduce cholesterol levels. An analysis of all double-blind trials in 1997 concluded that a daily amount of 10 grams of psyllium lowered cholesterol levels by 5 percent and LDL cholesterol by 9 percent. Adding, 5 to 10 grams of psyllium to your diet per day can lower cholesterol levels. Combining psyllium with oat bran may be even more effective.

Cordyceps sinensis, a fungus that contains glyconutrients can also prevent the accumulation of cholesterol deposits on blood vessel walls. It does so by suppressing blood lipid levels and by inhibiting LDL (bad cholesterol) oxidation by dangerous free radicals, which decreases areas of arterial damage. Stated simply, the sugars in cordyceps aid in the prevention of coronary artery disease.

Fucoidan from Brown Seaweed

Data from the Laboratory of Lipid Chemistry in Yokohama, Japan published in a 1999 issue of the *Journal of Nutrition* reveals that rats fed brown seaweed had significantly lower levels of blood fats that those who were not. After giving the rats seaweed for twenty-one days, scientists concluded that certain brown seaweed compounds (polysaccharides) work to alter the activity of enzymes in the liver that control the way fatty acids are metabolized, resulting in lower cholesterol levels in the blood.

The Anti-Clotting Action of Fucoidan

Several research studies have confirmed the ability of fucoidan to discourage the formation of blood clots. The most recent comes from the Department of Surgical Sciences in Stockholm, published in a November 2000 issue of the *European Journal of Vascular and Endovascular Surgery*. The scientists concluded that "Fucoidan is a more potent antiproliferative polysulphated polysaccharide than heparin." Heparin is a prescription blood thinner used to prevent blood clots, especially after surgery. Swedish doctors at Malmo University Hospital in Sweden also reported that fucoidan inhibits the formation of blood clots by preventing fibrin compounds from clumping and sticking to artery walls. The formation of blood clots can lead to heart attacks or strokes.

Other Supplements for Heart Health

Vitamin E
Scientific evidence supports the notion that the oxidation of LDL cholesterol is a risk factor in the development of coro-

nary artery disease. Vitamin E works as an antioxidant by preventing the oxidative damage that can lead to atherosclerosis. In one study, patients taking 1,600 mg/day of vitamin E recorded a 50 percent decrease in oxidative damage to LDL cholesterol. Of equal importance, a low blood level of vitamin E is considered an important risk factor in deaths from ischemic heart disease. Some experts even believe it has more impact than elevated cholesterol, high blood pressure or smoking. Another study found that people taking 100 IU of vitamin E or more daily had a substantial reduction in the progression of atherosclerosis.

Vitamin C

In a study conducted at UCLA, men who took 800 mg of vitamin C daily had a 42 percent reduction in mortality from cardiovascular disease, compared to men who only consumed the FDA Recommended Dietary Allowance (RDA) of 60 mg of vitamin C daily. In addition, men consuming the larger amounts of vitamin C lived an average of six years longer than the men who only consumed the RDA of 60 mg of vitamin C daily.

L-Carnitine

Studies report that carnitine can be therapeutically useful in the treatment of various forms of cardiovascular disease such as angina, heart attack, peripheral vascular disease, arrhythmia and high cholesterol. Carnitine also boosts energy delivery and use in muscles, and the heart is the most energy demanding "muscle" in the body.

Coenzyme Q10 (CoQ10)

Coenzyme Q10 functions as an antioxidant and participates in several enzymatic steps necessary for the generation of energy on a cellular level. It also has heart protective properties. In one double-blind study, patients with severe congestive heart failure who were given 150 mg per day of CoQ10 had a 38 percent decrease in hospitalizations due to worsening of heart failure compared to the control group.

Vitamins B6 and B12

Elevated levels of homocysteine are seen as a primary risk factor for cardiovascular disease. Vitamin B6 is necessary to convert homocysteine to cystathionine. Moreover, folic acid and vitamin B12 are required to convert homocysteine back to methionine. A deficiency of any one of these three B vitamins can lead to elevated homocysteine, which can predispose a person to heart disease.

Magnesium

Magnesium inhibits platelet aggregation by thinning the blood and relaxing blood vessels, which reduces the risk of developing a blood clot. Magnesium also boosts the oxygenation of the heart muscle by improving cardiac contractions. A magnesium deficiency has been associated with increased incidence of atherosclerosis, hypertension, strokes and heart attacks.

Omega-3 Fatty Acids

These fatty acids, when incorporated into the diet, appear to stabilize myocardial membranes, which reduces the risk of arrhythmia, thereby reducing the risk of sudden death. Higher doses of omega-3 fatty acids can also lower elevated serum triglyceride levels.

Potassium

People consuming diets containing foods that are high in potassium have a lower incidence of hypertension, which is directly associated with heart attacks and strokes. Several studies reveal that increasing potassium intake can lower blood pressure in individuals who have essential hypertension, and increasing dietary potassium can also enable a person with high blood pressure to reduce their medication.

Selenium

Low levels of selenium are considered significant risk factors for cardiovascular disease. Selenium is a powerful antioxidant that protects the heart. It also fights viral infections that may target the lining of the heart.

Soy Isoflavones

Genistein, one of the phytochemicals found in soy protein, inhibits the formation of blood clots and discourages the accumulation of cholesterol in blood vessels. It also has antioxidant properties and enhances the flexibility of arterial walls.

Hawthorn

Used extensively by doctors in Europe to treat cardiovascular and peripheral circulatory conditions, this herb helps to reduce blood pressure due to arteriosclerosis. It also appears to have the ability to regulate both low and high blood pressure. Its bioflavonoid content also helps to dilate both peripheral and coronary blood vessels explaining its use for angina.

Garlic

Garlic appears to lower bad cholesterol (LDL) while raising good cholesterol (HDL). It is also thought to prevent heart disease and atherosclerosis and discourage the formation of blood clots. The antioxidant effect in aged garlic has been reported to be beneficial in preventing stroke and arteriosclerosis.

Chapter Eleven

Glyconutrients, ADHD and Alzheimer's Disease

"Money is the most envied, but the least enjoyed. Health is the most enjoyed, but the least envied." *–Charles Caleb Colton*

If you have a child with ADHD (attention deficit hyperactivity disorder), you have lots of company. ADHD is the most frequently diagnosed psychiatric condition in children. Symptoms of ADHD include the inability to stay focused or to finish tasks, impulsive or aggressive behavior, distractibility and excessive movement even during sleep. Because kids will be kids, ADHD may go unrecognized until your child starts school.

The conventional treatment for ADHD is Ritalin (methylphenidate) or other similar drugs. Its seemingly casual and widespread use has caused considerable controversy and for good reason. The use of Ritalin for ADHD has increased by 700 percent over the last five years. In addition, reports show that the number of children under four taking the drug has almost tripled. The U.S. manufactures and consumes five times more Ritalin than the rest of the world combined. In fact, in 1996, the World Health Organization warned that Ritalin overuse had reached dangerous proportions.

While it seems crazy, in some people with ADHD the stimulant properties of Ritalin work to calm rather than excite. Ritalin is not without significant side effects, however, and can cause dependency and possible drug abuse. Furthermore, putting your already rambunctious child on an amphetamine-like drug warrants concern. You need to check out the possibility that a nutrient deficiency may be the real cause behind your child's behavior.

Bad Sugars and ADHD

Parents who live with ADHD are only too familiar with the link between white sugar and behavior. Children with ADHD often react with extreme behavior after eating sweets, suggesting that their ability to properly metabolize sugar may be impaired. In addition, miscommunication between glycoproteins may be at the heart of the problem. Many experts believe that children with ADHD fail to digest sucrose (white sugar) properly, suggesting that they may lack the right enzymes needed to synthesize glyconutrients from glucose.

In a study published in the January/March 1998 issue of *Integrative and Physiological and Behavioral Science*, researchers tested seventeen children who had been diagnosed with ADHD. For three weeks, a glyconutrient supplement that included all of the eight major glyconutrients was given. After that time period, another plant-derived supplement was added. The authors of the study concluded "Most important, the dietary supplements we used significantly reduced the number and severity of ADHD symptoms of children, whether they were taking or not taking methylphenidate." In another study published in a recent issue of *Proceedings of the Fisher Institute for Medical Research*, researchers concluded that the essential eight sugars improved the health of ADHD subjects and reduced the number and severity of symptoms.

Antibiotics and Ear Infections in Children

Here's another reason to use antibiotics judiciously. Repeated antibiotic therapy causes a growth of dysbiotic flora in the bowel that destroys friendly bacteria. Consequently, the immune system is weakened and yeast organisms can grow. Both food allergies and ADHD have been linked to fungal infections. Laboratory tests show high levels of fungal metabolites in children with ADHD. Of equal interest is the existing link between the number of childhood inner ear infections and hyperactive behavior, emphasizing the impact of early antibiotics use. Using a good probiotic or acidophilus supplement for four to six months after antibiotic therapy can help prevent these health risks.

Your child may also be suffering from a lack of EFAs (essential fatty acids). Fatty acids are vital for proper brain development and function, and many children with ADHD have trouble processing fats into fatty acids. It's no coincidence that hyperactive kids are also prone to eczema, allergies, and asthma—all of which are linked to low EFAs. Moreover, low levels of the omega-3 fatty acids corresponded to more temper tantrums, learning disabilities and even sleep disorders. Omega-3 EFAs are found in flaxseed, safflower and fish oils.

The Magnesium Factor and ADHD

The mineral that is most lacking in children with ADHD is magnesium. Of 116 children with ADHD, a magnesium deficiency was found in 95 percent of those tested. In another study, fifty children who had ADHD and low magnesium levels who were given 200 mg of magnesium daily for six months experienced significant improvement. Guess what foods are rich in magnesium—fresh fruits and vegetables, not potato chips and Ding Dongs.

Learning Disorders and Brain Cell Molecules

While glucose provides brain fuel, glycoproteins enable the brain to operate at maximum efficiency. For this reason, making sure that a wide array of glyconutrients, or brain building blocks, are continually supplied only makes good sense. In one study of an eight-year-old boy with dyslexia published in the August 1997 supplemental issue of the *Journal of the American Nutraceutical Industry*, a combination of glyconutrients and other phytochemicals (plant chemicals) resulted in an advance from low to middle-level school performance. It was also noted that the child was less agitated and frustrated.

Alzheimer's Disease and Sugars

Approximately four million Americans have Alzheimer's disease today; and with baby boomers entering the golden years, it's estimated that fourteen million will have it by the mid twenty-first century. Alzheimer's is a degenerative disease that causes the transformation of healthy brain tissue into twisted, spaghetti-like masses called neurofibrillary tangles. The cause of Alzheimer's remains unknown. Everything from aluminum ingestion to malnutrition has been implicated. When the disease is in its early stages, drugs called ACE inhibitors are used to help inhibit memory loss and enhance mental function. Unfortunately, these drugs work for a maximum of three years after diagnosis.

Glucose is the brain's sole source of fuel. If blood glucose levels dip, so does our ability to think. Interestingly, in a 1994 issue of *Gerontology*, scientists reported that brain cells of test subjects with Alzheimer's disease had a serious problem metabolizing glucose. In another report published in 1993 in the *Journal of Internal Medicine*, consistently low levels of blood glucose were also associated with Alzheimer's disease. Fucose, galactose and N-acetylneuraminic acid supplementation have all been associated with better memory recall. In fact, in animal studies conducted at La Trobe University in Australia, fucose was actually able to overcome artificially induced amnesia.

Other Supplements that Improve Brain Function

Choline

Because Alzheimer's impacts cholinergic neurons in the cerebral cortex of the brain, choline may be of value. The activity of these particular neurons is profoundly affected by a neurotransmitter called acetylcholine. The enzyme that produces acetylcholine can be faulty in people with Alzheimer's, resulting in low levels of this vital neurotransmitter.

Phosphatidylserine

Phospholipids are substances that make up the structural framework of cell membranes, and those found in the brain are loaded with phosphatidylserine. In one study, fifty-one people with early-stage Alzheimer's disease either took a phosphatidylserine supplement or a placebo every day for four months. Those on the supplement improved in multiple areas of mental function and performance. Other studies show that people with senile dementia who took phosphatidylserine for sixty days displayed improved memory and mental ability. Interestingly, these positive effects continued even after they discontinued supplementation.

Acetyl-L-Carnitine (ALC)

This amino acid facilitates the conversion of fat into energy and also works to clear waste products created from fat metabolism. L-carnitine and its cousin, acetyl-L-carnitine, have shown usefulness in the treatment of Alzheimer's disease and dementia. Acetyl-L-carnitine is also a precursor for acetylcholine, which, as previously mentioned, is innately involved in brain function. Acetyl-L-carnitine may help slow the degeneration of brain cells seen in Alzheimer's disease.

Vitamin E

Vitamin E is a stellar antioxidant, which helps prevent brain cell damage. In one clinical trial, a group of people with moderate Alzheimer's who were placed on vitamin E daily showed a slowing of mental and psychological decline typically seen in the disease. Of equal importance, another long-term study suggests that vitamin E may substantially lower the risk of developing Alzheimer's disease.

Vitamin C

Having a deficiency of vitamin C has been observed in people with Alzheimer's. In fact, those that had the lowest levels also had the most serious decline in mental function. The link is thought to involve the brain cell damage of free radicals that takes place during the progression of Alzheimer's. The more free radicals you have, the more vitamin C you need.

Ginkgo biloba

This famous brain boosting herb can benefit anyone with Alzheimer's disease by rounding up dangerous free radicals, by discouraging the formation of clots and most importantly by enhancing the delivery of oxygen and nutrients to brain cells. There is some data that shows the ability of ginkgo improves function of cholinergic neurons that are targeted by the disease. Several studies suggest that ginkgo may reverse the effects of aging on the brain which would decrease senility and may even slow the onset of Alzheimer's disease.

Huperzine A

Huperzine A is an extract taken from a moss plant that may improve memory and learning capacity. Huperzine A inhibits an enzyme in the body that breaks down acetylcholine, which is directly involved in memory and learning processes. For this reason, it may hold potential benefits for people with Alzheimer's disease.

Vinpocetine

Vinpocetine is a synthetically created product derived from vincamine, a substance found in the periwinkle (*Vinca minor*) plant. European practitioners have used vinpocetine to alleviate symptoms caused by compromised brain circulation. Vinpocetine boosts circulation and, therefore, oxygenation of brain cells by relaxing blood vessels found in the brain. It also has significant antioxidant actions. Several studies confirm its ability to enhance memory and mental performance in people with mild dementia.

Chapter Twelve

Chronic Fatigue, Fibromyalgia and Other Syndromes

"The health of the people is really the foundation upon which all their happiness and all their powers as a state depend." *–Benjamin Disraeli*

A *syndrome* is nothing more than a word to describe a disease that no one really understands. Chronic fatigue syndrome (CFS) is such a disease and is characterized by debilitating fatigue and a variety of other complaints. It affects eight hundred thousand Americans and is three times more common in women. It is thought that over 85 percent of people with CFS go undiagnosed, and as a result, don't receive proper medical care for their illness.

Symptoms of CFS can range from persistent or recurring sore throat, tender lymph nodes, muscle pain, joint pain, headaches, poor sleep and debilitating fatigue. Interestingly, people with CFS appear to have dysfunctional immunity across the board. Not surprisingly, they also lack the very sugars this book has focused on. In a test study conducted at the University of California at Irvine, researchers found that the people with CFS had much lower glyconutrient activity, as well as lower natural killer cell counts.

People with CFS and the Essential Eight Sugars

We already know that the addition of supplemental sugars not only stimulates glycoprotein performance, but also increases the number of natural killer cell levels, stops premature cell death, and gives the immune system what might be called an "overhaul." One study on the essential eight sugars discussed earlier, found that eight monosaccharides are required for the synthesis of glycoproteins. They found that adding these sugars improved abnormal immune functions (in vitro) in blood samples of patients with CFS.

Cordyceps sinensis and Reishi Mushrooms

Cordyceps is a unique black mushroom that has been traditionally used to increase energy and endurance in Asia. It contains a number of healing sugars and has been used to fight infection, respiratory disorders and cancer. Its singular tonic action makes it a perfect choice for people with CFS. In addition, another mushroom called reishi contains highly active polysaccharides that also work to reinvigorate a weakened immune system. The sugar compounds found in both of these mushrooms also fight viral infections—something that may be driving CFS.

Nicotinamide Adenine Dinucleotide (NADH)

NADH was studied in a double-blind study in a group of people with chronic fatigue syndrome. Twenty-six subjects were randomly assigned to receive either 10 mg of NADH or placebo for a four-week period. The data showed that eight of twenty-six patients responded favorably to NADH, while only two of twenty-six test subjects taking the placebo improved.

Magnesium

Some studies suggest that individuals with chronic fatigue syndrome have lower red cell magnesium concentrations. Some patients treated with magnesium have better energy levels, better moods and less pain.

Omega-3 and Omega-6 Fatty Acids

Another study of a group of people that had suffered from CFS for years found that giving them a supplement with linolenic, gamma-linolenic, eicosapentaenoic and docosahexaenoic acids resulted in improvement in the majority of test subjects. The study actually suggests that essential fatty acid supplementation should be considered for anyone with chronic fatigue syndrome.

Folic Acid

Substantial data points to low folic acid levels in people with chronic fatigue syndrome. Naturally, the assumption that raising those levels may benefit CFS sufferers is worth considering.

Fibromyalgia

Fibromyalgia, another mystifying disease that had no name twenty years ago, affects three to six million people. Fibromyalgia primarily targets women of childbearing age and has been linked to various disorders. The most prominent symptom of fibromyalgia is widespread muscle and skeletal pain that often occurs in a number of trigger points found throughout the body. Other symptoms that commonly occur include disturbed sleep patterns, morning stiffness, depression, recurrent headaches, constipation, racing heart beats and allergies. Interestingly, fibromyalgia often accompanies other diseases such as chronic fatigue syndrome and irritable bowel syndrome. The pain of fibromyalgia fails to respond well to anti-inflammatory drugs such as NSAIDs, aspirin and corticosteroids. The use of antidepressants has brought some relief, but the disease continues to elude successful treatment.

The Sugar Link to Fibromyalgia

Impaired muscle cell repair and regeneration has been strongly linked to fibromyalgia. Mannose prompts the restoration of tissue and promotes better reception of hormones in the body. In addition, because low serotonin levels may play a role in this disease the use of glyconutrients such as mannose positively impact the way brain chemicals are produced and used. In fact, tests have found that when glyconutrients are taken away from certain brain chemicals, their uptake by surrounding cells is decreased.

Fibromyalgia may also be linked to a hidden virus—a fact that may signal weakened immune function. If so, glyconutrient supplementation can work to eradicate hidden viral infections. Glucosamine may also be of benefit for its analgesic action in controlling pain.

In a study published in the January/March issue of *Integrative and Physiological and Behavioral Science*, a group of test subjects with fibromyalgia and chronic fatigue syndrome who consumed a nutritional supplement containing freeze-dried aloe vera extract (rich in acetylated mannans) and other natural compounds reported marked significant improvement in their symptoms.

S-Adenosylmethionine (SAMe)

S-adenosylmethionine exerts a natural anti-inflammatory, analgesic and antidepressant effect. One study showed that forty-four people with fibromyalgia reported the improvements in their symptoms after taking SAMe. Moreover, other test subjects also found that SAMe supplementation reduced depression, as well as the number of trigger points.

5-Hydroxytryptophan (5-HTP)

Because so many people with fibromyalgia have abnormal serotonin metabolic pathways, using natural compounds that stimulate the protection of serotonin only makes sense. The amino acid tryptophan and 5-hydroxytryptophan (5-HTP) both raise serotonin activity. When used in studies for the treatment of fibromyalgia, test subjects reported improvements in depression, anxiety, insomnia and muscle aches.

Magnesium and Malic Acid

Using both of these compounds together can result in a significant decrease in pain among people with fibromyalgia, and symptoms of fatigue have also improved. Magnesium and malic acid exert oxygen-sparing effects, so if you're low in either one, you can suffer from a lack of cellular oxygen in muscle tissue, which can cause chronic pain. Magnesium and malic acid also reduce lactic acid levels in muscle tissue. Lactic acid causes muscle soreness after strenuous exercise.

Vitamin B1 (Thiamin)

Symptoms of a thiamin deficiency are quite similar to those of fibromyalgia (fatigue, depression, confusion, numbness or tingling, the hands and feet, shortness of breath, among others).

Astragalus

The Chinese have valued astragalus for centuries for its immune-enhancing and adaptogenic properties. As an adaptogen, it may modify and improve the body's response to stress through action on the adrenal cortex. Astragalus enhances the effects of interferon and may increase cellular oxygenation of the heart and cerebrovascular tissue and improve stamina and endurance.

Failure to Thrive and Wasting Syndromes

Considered one of the most tragic of childhood diseases, Failure to thrive syndrome (FTT), as well as its cousin cachexia, causes the body to literally waste away. Seen in adults in cases of AIDS or cancer, both disorders have been linked with the inability of the body to use dietary nutrients. According to a report in the January 1993 *Journal of Pediatrics*, carbohydrate-deficient glycoproteins were found in five children who failed to thrive during their first year of life.

Research data indicates that supplementing the diets of children who have FTT with glyconutrients resulted in a significant improvement in symptoms. It appears that a direct cause of FTT symptoms is the failure of glycoproteins to transport sugar, something that can actually start in the placenta. This malfunction of glucose transporters, or glycoproteins, can occur not only in the placenta, but in the blood-brain barrier and muscle cells of the developing infant as well. When this occurs, an important energy source becomes unavailable resulting in a whole host of undesirable symptoms including seizures and delayed development. You don't have to be a rocket scientist to understand that compromised glucose transport impacts virtually every body system. Moreover, the inability to metabolize certain sugars due to genetic enzyme deficiencies can also result in wasting, retarded growth and impaired immune function. Apparently, mannose, galactose, fucose and N-acetylneuraminic acid are all involved and experts have concluded that because these sugar molecules play such a crucial role in functions involving FTT, their supplementation may be of great value.

Chapter Thirteen

Glyconutrients as Infection Busters

"The groundwork of all happiness is health." –*Leigh Hunt*

Immune cells aren't the only cells with sugar components on their surfaces. Infectious organisms also have sugar molecules on their surfaces, and when they enter the body, all kinds of chattering between friend and foe cells occurs and the fight begins. The entire premise of this book is that the availability of various glyconutrients such as mannose, fucose or polysaccharide K to immune cells supplies the raw materials that enables them to interrupt the process of infection. How do they accomplish this? By slowing down the reproduction of disease organisms and by boosting immune cell activity (especially macrophages).

We've already talked about the role of glycoproteins in immunity—they are the molecules ultimately responsible for telling white blood cells where to migrate for their attack. And we've already documented the studies showing that mannose significantly boosts the action of the white blood cells that destroy pathogens and antibodies in the bloodstream.

In a time when more clever and evasive microbes threaten us worldwide, using glyconutrients to prevent and control infections is crucial.

Antibiotic Resistance: A Good Thing Gone Bad

Bacterial resistance to antibiotics is a growing public health threat. It's as simple as that. Drugs that were considered magic bullets for bacterial infections have now created super bugs that pose a very serious health threat for all. Bacteria are fighting back by mutating into forms that resist even our most potent antibiotics. The implications are frightening. The appearance of flesh-eating bacteria or penicillin-resistant strep over the last few years illustrates just how smart these microbes are becoming. Some experts warn that we are currently only one antibiotic away from a major infectious epidemic that won't respond to anything in our antibiotic arsenal. New reports reveal that a minimum of 70 percent of the bacteria that cause hospital-acquired infections are resistant to at least one antibiotic.

How did this microbe disaster happen? It has been the direct result of the over-prescription of antibiotic drugs for everything from a cold to a hangnail. In fact, the Centers for Disease Control and Prevention (CDC) estimate that one hundred million courses of antibiotics are provided by office-based doctors each year. In 1954, two million pounds of antibiotics were produced in the United States. Today, that figure exceeds fifty million pounds.

Most experts agree that many antibiotic prescriptions are unnecessary, and many put that number as high as 50 percent. Remember that antibiotics are only effective against bacteria. They are completely useless against the viruses that cause colds, flus and some sore throats. Moreover, not taking an antibiotic medicine long enough has also created the formation of super bugs. Most of us don't want to keep taking a medicine if we feel fine, but completing a full course of antibiotics is vital for the total eradication of a bacteria from the body. The misuse of these life-saving drugs has made it harder to get rid of common conditions like sinusitis and has nearly doubled the incidence of bacteria-caused upper respiratory infections over the last twenty years. Side effects of prolonged or repeated antibiotic use include yeast infections and the loss of friendly flora in the intestines, which can compromise immunity and even stimulate allergies or contribute to behavioral disorders like ADHD.

Antibiotic abuse has transformed what were curable germs into new antibiotic-resistant bacteria. While antibiotics are certainly warranted for serious infections, the plant kingdom also provides natural saccharides (sugars) that stimulate our immune systems to successfully defeat infectious invaders. Before penicillin was discovered, herbs like echinacea were readily prescribed for infections by eclectic physicians of the late nineteenth century. In the wake of the current antibiotic crisis, our best option is to take them more judiciously and to maximize our own immune defenses.

Sugar-Coated Bacteria

Bacteria (normally treated with antibiotics) have sugar-bound proteins called adhesins that stick to the sugar portion of our cells and vice versa. This "sticking" is considered the first step in the process of a bacterial invasion. Research experts point out that bacteria with the ability to engage in this exchange include *E. coli, N. gonorrhea, Mycobacterium tuberculosis*, and some strains of salmonella and staphylococci. A defect in the molecules could impede this "sticky sugar" interaction. Acemannan (a derivative of mannose) has proven antimicrobial actions.

Glyconutrients fight bacteria in two vital ways. They keep bacteria from reproducing and colonizing, and they potentiate immune cell defense capabilities.

Echinacea Polysaccharides

Echinacea, also known as purple coneflower, has been used for generations by Native Americans for its impressive natural antibiotic action. Echinacea stimulates the production of immune natural killer cells and destroys a broad range of disease-causing bacteria. Echinacea can be a boon to the elderly who are susceptible to bacterial infections. A new study conducted by scientists at McGill University in Montreal, Canada showed that two weeks of supplementation with echinacea rejuvenated the production of immune killer cells even in animals of advanced age. Newly published findings show that echinacea extracts are potent activators of natural killer cells enabling them to target and break up bacteria. Ideally, it's best to use echinacea in two-week intervals as a preventive agent or to take it during the initial stages of an infection. If you're already sick, maximum stimulation from echinacea occurs between three to six days after the first dose; so it needs to be taken at the first sign of an infection. Be aware that the immune-regulating polysaccharides found in echinacea are not viable when placed in alcohol. Alcohol extracts destroy the polysaccharide content of echinacea, therefore removing its immune-regulating properties.

Mannose, Fucose and Beta-Glucans

Mannose and fucose have the ability to kill bacteria and to help fortify our resistance to infection. New studies reveal that because bacteria have lectins on their surface that stick to mannose receptors on the surface of their host, supplying the body with mannose can help deflect host binding so an infection can be either foiled or lessened. The mannose binds to the bacteria keeping it from infecting healthy tissue receptors. Mannose has been shown to prevent this binding in several kinds of bacteria including *Salmonella typhimurium* and *Escherichia coli* (*E. coli*). Interestingly, xylose was able to kill candida and gram-negative bacteria. Studies also tell us that fucose works to inhibit the adhesion of bacteria to respiratory cells and can actually reverse some infectious processes. A review of literature on beta-glucans and immune function reveals that these sugars also stimulate macrophages and can also prevent infection by boosting natural killer cell activity, and by stimulating the action of an enzyme that breaks bacterial cells open.

Arabinogalactans

These glyconutrients are found in the bark of some trees and other fibrous foods. Studies confirm that they improve the body's immunity by boosting the activity of the natural killer (NK) cells. Consequently, these sugars play a vital role in building resistance to both bacterial and viral invaders. Arabinogalactans dramatically enhance macrophage activity and also inhibit bacteria from attaching to cells. Moreover, it helps to increase friendly probiotic activity by prompting the formation of good bacteria such as lactobacillus and bifidobacteria.

A Note on Ear Infections

According to the World Health Organization, antibiotic-resistant bacteria are due, in part, to the over-prescription and misuse of antibiotics for one of the most troublesome child-hood illnesses—ear infections. To make matters worse, ear infections are increasing and the use of new and more power-ful drugs are failing to control their recurrence.

Studies strongly suggest that using mannose can help inhibit the progress of an ear infection. In fact, one study published in a recent issue of *Molecular and Cellular Biochemistry* reported that using mannose in combination with antibiotics was better than antibiotic treatment alone. According to another report found in the December 2000 issue of *Vaccine*, using xylitol dramatically reduced the number of ear infections in children by inhibiting the growth and attachment of *Streptococcus pneumoniae* in the tubes that run from the throat to the ear. If your child has multiple ear infections annually, consider assessing their immune system.

Xylitol and Ear Infections

A study published in the 1996 issue of the *British Medical Journal* reported a trial that involved over 306 children with a history of ear infections. Half of the children chewed xyli-tol-containing gum at a rate of two pieces several times daily after meals and snacks. The other half chewed ordinary gum. Over a sixty day period, 21 percent of the regular gum chewers as opposed to 12 percent of the xylitol group, came down with one or more ear infections. Interestingly, just chewing gum seems to prevent ear infections by clearing fluid from the ear canals; however, the presence of white sugar in the gum may also stimulate the growth of bacteria. The xylitol-chewing children experienced almost a 50 per-cent drop in ear infections because it not only kept fluid flowing in the ear canals, it inhibited the growth of infec-tious bacteria.

Although xylitol is considered safe, it can cause diarrhea. If you're using it to sweeten foods in granular form, you may have to adjust your dosages until the bowel adapts.

Urinary Tract Infections

As one of the most common bacterial infections seen today, urinary tract infections (UTIs) account for seven million patient visits annually, and it's estimated that 20 percent of women will suffer with symptoms of a urinary tract infection some time in their lives. A UTI is typically treated with potent antibiotic drugs. Most cases are caused by the contamination of the urinary tract by *E. coli* bacteria. *E. coli* bacteria have sugar molecules that enable them to stick to the cells that occupy the lining of the bladder. There is evidence that a combination of mannose and glucose sugars was able to reduce the severity of a urinary tract infection within twenty-four hours. Interestingly, mannose is found in cranberry juice, which is also very highly recommended for urinary tract infections.

Yeast (Candida) Infections

While more research is needed on the workings of sugars and fungi, we do know that yeast (*Candida albicans*) infections interact with our body cells through the action of mannose-containing proteins found on their surface. Scientists announced in the April 2003 issue of the *International Journal of Immunopharmacology* that mannose does indeed speed up the destruction of yeast organisms.

Like other infectious invaders, macrophages bind to the mannose molecules found on candida. In one study conducted at the Department of Botany and Microbiology at the University of Kuwait, the addition of mannose and N-acetylglucosamine was so significant that it protected laboratory test mice against the reproduction of yeast in the digestive tract. Our ability to fight other fungal infections such as athlete's foot and nail fungus may also be enhanced through glyconutrient stimulation.

Viral Diseases

Even with all of our sophisticated drugs, viruses have managed to evade destruction. More than four hundred viruses are known to infect human cells. Like bacteria and fungi, viruses also have glycoproteins that reside on their surfaces. For example, the influenza virus has a sugar compound that helps it pierce the membrane of a healthy human cell and set up housekeeping. In the August 2000 issue of the *Journal of Immunology*, mannose sugars bound to compounds called lectins, which were found to be formidable virus hunters. Remember that some viruses like herpes can stay dormant and hide in our cells for years and can surface from time to time when our immune defenses become weakened due to stress.

The Cold and Flu Scourge

Cold and flu bugs are poised and ready to attack, and the projected casualty count for this year numbers in the millions. Together, this viral duo conspire to cause more missed days at school and in the workplace than any other ailment. Flu alone accounts for 192 million days spent in bed every year. Most adults catch an average of three colds each year, and children catch considerably more. Viruses coat telephones, stick to money, inhabit coffee cups and love to travel from hand to hand in tiny droplets. Rightly referred to as microbial terrorists, they take healthy cells hostage, hijack their protein-making machinery, replicate themselves, and then start the process all over again in another cell. In addition, viruses are shape shifters that periodically mutate so our army of antibodies has a hard time keeping up.

Once inside the body, viruses trigger immune responses (fever, excess mucus, sneezing, and coughing, among others). Conventional therapies are designed to suppress these symptoms: a practice that has contributed to the overuse of antibiotics, antihistamines and pain killing drugs. Unlike bacteria, viruses are not destroyed by antibiotics. According to a report in a recent issue of the *Journal of Clinical Microbiology*, over 50 percent of colds are needlessly treated with antibiotics. Antihistamines can cause nasal passages to become abnormally dry, creating an even more hospitable environment for infectious organisms to grow. These drugs have also been linked to increases in blood pressure and anxiety.

The flu and its complications can pose a serious threat for the elderly, who can develop life-threatening diseases like pneumonia. Inactivity and nutrient depletion commonly seen in older populations increase the risk of respiratory infection due to weakened immunity. The same is true of people with heart disease and other chronic illnesses. In all, twenty thousand people die every year from flu-related illnesses.

The Role of Sugars in Viral Infection

Cold and flu viruses have the distinct ability to enter a healthy cell by initially binding with the sugar sialic acid, which inhabits the cell surface of a human glycoprotein. When the virus' cellular structure adheres to this sugar, the lock to the cell door is opened and the virus is allowed to enter and replicate itself at a rapid rate. When a new virus is formed, it must leave its host cell. In order to succeed, the virus has to break through a sugar coating. Interestingly, it releases sugar-dissolving enzymes enabling it to break free and start the process all over again. Using medicinal compounds that inhibit the action of this enzyme could certainly shorten the duration of a bout with the flu.

Scientists at the Biomolecular Research Institute in Victoria Australia reported in the April 2001 issue of *Protein Science* that N-acetylneuraminic acid was an antiflu virus agent. Another study suggests that it may be a very effective flu treatment if given early enough. Like bacteria, flu viruses continually mutate so each year our immune systems have to deal with a whole new viral ball game.

One animal study published in a 1995 issue of *Antimicrobial Agents and Chemotherapy* reported that a N-acetylneuraminic acid mixture was up to one thousand times more effective in fighting the influenza virus than potent antiviral drugs. Viruses also cause cold sores (herpes), hepatitis, viral pneumonia, and the common cold. In addition, scientists actually administered the sugar, N-acetylneuramine through an inhaler to laboratory test animals with bronchitis and concluded that it helped to minimize the infection. Many glyconutrients exert antiviral activity because they stimulate macrophages to release a powerful immune weapon called interferon. As stated earlier, they also interfere with viral function and replication.

AIDS, Aloe and Antibody Attack

Glycoproteins are critically important in the study of AIDS. Recent studies confirm that sugars may play a major role in how the AIDS virus spreads. Japanese researchers at the AIDS Research Center in Tokyo have found that mannose, fucose and acetylglucosamine actually inhibited the HIV virus. In addition, according to a study in a 1990 issue of the *American Journal of Clinical Nutrition*, a xylose deficiency was found in

AIDS patients suggesting that xylose supplementation may boost better energy levels.

In a study published in a 2000 issue of *Phytotherapy Research* and conducted at the Department of Microbiology at the University of Texas at Antonio, researchers reported that mannose from aloe vera showed significant activity against the Coxsackie virus by dramatically boosting antibody attack. In fact, they concluded that aloe polymannose can "potentiate" antibody production against not only these viruses but also against other difficult viruses like herpes as well. And when it comes to stubborn parasitic infections, two sugars shine. The amoebal parasite called acanthamoeba can cause serious eye infections; and like *E. coli*, it sticks to mannose receptors on healthy cells. We know that mannose and N-acetyl-d-glucosamine can inhibit amoeba-induced infections.

Other Immune-Boosting Agents

Zinc

Human clinical trials on the use of zinc in viral infections such as colds and influenza indicate that zinc gluconate lozenges may be effective in reducing the duration and severity of symptoms. In several randomized, controlled trials, it was determined that zinc gluconate lozenges have a therapeutic effect in treating the common cold; they also boost immune defenses against both bacterial and viral infections. Nasal sprays that contain zinc also have a good track record. Zinc sprays can prevent rhinoviruses from attaching to the mucus membranes in your nose.

Vitamin A

The antioxidant actions of vitamin A help facilitate the toxic waste removal that must occur when infectious organisms invade the body. Vitamin A also stimulates the action of immune cells and works well with other immune-boosting supplements.

Elderberry

Elderberry gained its flu-fighting fame from a 1995 double-blind, placebo-controlled study of forty patients with influenza published in the *Journal of Alternative and Complementary Medicine*. Researchers found that 90 percent of those with the flu who took 10 ml of elderberry extract (sambucol) four times daily were completely symptom free after only three days.

Apparently, elderberry extract elevates immune proteins called cytokines. Elderberry's ability to block the action of an enzyme called neuraminidase, however, is what has the scientific community buzzing. Neuraminidase allows flu viruses to pop through healthy cell membranes and reproduce. Blocking neuraminidase goes a long way in slowing down a tough flu virus.

Vitamin C and Calcium

A recent study confirms that taking vitamin C both prevents and relieves symptoms of the common cold. In the study, groups took hourly doses of 1,000 mg of vitamin C for the first six hours and then three times daily thereafter. Calcium is essential for the production of white blood cells and plays a vital role in the absorption of vitamin C.

Goldenseal

Goldenseal contains a powerful antimicrobial compound called berberine, which is often coupled with echinacea to maximize each herb's antimicrobial effect.

Combinations of goldenseal and echinacea are one of the leading selling herbal supplements in the U.S. Berberine has many documented antimicrobial activities and is often used to treat bacterial gastrointestinal infections.

Astragalus

Studies have reported that astragalus promotes regeneration of cells in the lungs after a bout with bronchitis. It also enhances the effects of interferon and may act not only to improve resistance to viral infections, but also to decrease their duration.

Chapter Fourteen

Other Stellar Immune Boosters

"Take care of your body with steadfast fidelity. The soul must see through these eyes alone, and if they are dim, the whole world is clouded."
—Johann Wolfgang Von Goethe

While the focus of this book has been on the immune-boosting powers of glyconutrients, this chapter focuses on other remarkable immune boosting substances that can be combined with glyconutrient therapy to strengthen or normalize the immune system. These supplements are my personal favorites because they are tried and true and contribute to maximum disease resistance. For me, glyconutrients and the following compounds are invaluable supplements that should be used by everyone, especially in light of the new and varied immune threats we face today. Their application can make the difference between disease vulnerability and disease resistance.

Transfer Factors: Evidence-Based Medicine

In 1976, researcher H. Sherwood Lawrence saw the potential of transfer factors (TF) for people with serious autoimmune disorders. Today, transfer factors are used to treat various autoimmune conditions because they serve to modulate and normalize immune response. Simply stated, by taking TFs, we borrow immune memory from a compatible source (immune boosted eggs or cow colostrum), which has already experienced hundreds of infectious organisms. So when we encounter any of these organisms, we have a profound advantage.

To date, over three thousand clinical studies and papers have been published on transfer factors. Scores of well-respected international scientists and physicians have established the effectiveness and safety of transfer factors. Transfer factors are tiny immune messenger molecules—a sequence of amino acids that impart immune signals between immune cells. Transfer factors educate naive cells to single out invaders more quickly. They work to provide T lymphocyte cells with a blueprint and immune markers that act as guides to mount a swift attack, cutting down the time they take to fight infection. In addition, transfer factors help the immune system widen its storehouse of antibodies, which helps to expand immune memory to better remember and deal with future infections.

Bug-Busting Garlic

No natural antibiotic list would be complete without the garlic clove. Garlic was used by Albert Schweitzer to treat dysentery in Africa, and Russians turned to garlic when their supplies of penicillin dwindled. Allicin is what gives garlic its broad-spectrum antibiotic punch. Apparently, garlic adds much more than taste to food. Scientists at the Department of Bacteriology at the Hirosaki University School of Medicine recently discovered that garlic powder may actually prevent bacteria-caused food poisoning from *E. coli* and salmonella contamination. And, if that wasn't good enough, researchers at the Weizmann Institute of Science in Israel reported that allicin fights against a wide range of gram-negative and gram-positive bacteria, including multi-drug-resistant strains.

Garlic is a powerful immune booster that stimulates the multiplication of infection-fighting white cells, boosts natural killer cell activity, and increases the efficiency of antibody production. And people who eat a lot of garlic have less incidence of bowel cancer.

St. John's Wort Fights Infection

Surprisingly, this well-known natural antidepressant has powerful antibacterial properties. The *Lancet* recently reported that the hyperforin content of St. John's wort has potent antibacterial properties. German scientists looked at its effect against the growth of various bacteria and on *Candida albicans* (the fungus that causes thrush). They discovered that relatively small doses of St. John's wort inhibited the growth of certain bacteria that had become resistant to penicillin and did so with no toxic side effects. Their research validates the use of St. John's wort on infected wounds and rashes during the middle ages. Look for St. John's wort products with a standardized 0.3 percent hypericin content.

Berberine's Natural Antibiotic Punch

Herbs like goldenseal and goldenthread contain a powerful microbe-killing alkaloid called berberine. This year, scientists from the Biotechnology Center at Tufts University in Medford, Massachusetts reported that berberine inhibited the growth of a very resistant strain of staphylococcus. Staph infections are difficult to treat by any standards. In addition, an article in the April 2000 issue of *Alternative Medicine Review* stated that berberine extracts have significant antimicrobial activity against bacteria, viruses and fungi. Berberine-containing herbs are particularly good for bacterial diarrhea, intestinal parasites, and for bladder and eye infections.

Elderberry: Enzymatic Blocker

This herb (also commonly called "sambucol," a standardized black elderberry extract) has potent antiviral properties. Its ability to block the action of an enzyme called neuraminidase is key in its ability to fight viral infections. Neuraminidase allows flu viruses to pop through healthy cell membranes and reproduce. Inhibiting this enzyme helps to stop the spread of viruses and can significantly shorten the duration of the flu. Ironically, medical scientists have taken a cue from nature and are developing synthetic neuraminidase inhibitors.

In 1995, a double-blind placebo-controlled study of forty patients with influenza published in the *Journal of Alternative and Complementary Medicine* found that 90 percent of those with the flu who took 10 ml of elderberry extract (Sambucol) four times daily were completely symptom-free after only three days. Apparently, elderberry extract elevates immune proteins called cytokines, which destroy invading pathogens. This is bad news for viruses because cytokines prevent viral replication. If you already have the flu, triple the dosage. Elderberry syrup, by the way, is delicious and very user-friendly for children.

Out-of-the-Ordinary Olive Leaf

The olive tree isn't only famous for its fruit and oil, its leaves contain marvelous compounds that help to rebuild the immune system. Olive leaf extract has proven natural antibiotic actions against bacteria, fungi, yeast and parasites. One of its chemical constituents called oleuropein is a bitter glucoside and is thought to be responsible for its ability to fight both infectious and degenerative diseases. Moreover olive leaf may lessen the duration of a viral infection by interfering with its replication, thereby preventing the virus from spreading to new host cells. Olive leaf may also reduce high blood pressure.

Vitamin C Has Immune Clout

A recent study found that vitamin C worked to both prevent and relieve symptoms of a viral respiratory infection in groups who took hourly doses of 1,000 mg for the first six hours and then three times daily thereafter. Reported flu and cold symptoms in the test group decreased 85 percent compared with the control group. And laboratory tests suggest that flu viruses are ten thousand times as infective if your vitamin C levels are low. Vitamin C increases the production of infection-fighting white blood cells and antibodies and boosts the levels of interferon, which coats and guards the surface of cells from viral invasion. The key is to take doses of vitamin C frequently. Keep in mind that mega-doses of vitamin C can cause diarrhea.

Bioflavonoids Battle the Bugs

These compounds complement vitamin C and protect the body against damage from environmental pollutants and microbial invaders by preventing toxic molecules from attaching to cell membranes. Bioflavonoids help to compete with foreign substances or microbes by parking themselves on cell receptor sites. As a result, the dangerous invader cannot. Bioflavonoids are abundantly found in fresh vegetables and fruits and support the notion that plant and fruit phytonutrients protect us from disease.

Zinc Germ Zappers

Zinc should be added to everyone's armory of antiviral compounds. Zinc prevents rhinoviruses from attaching to the mucus membranes in your nose. This year, scientists at the Immunology Center in Ancona, Italy reported that the molecular structures found in zinc are what maintain our immune response to disease. The study concluded that dietary supplementation with zinc for between one and two months decreases the incidence of infection and increases the survival rate following infection in older individuals. In other clinical trials, zinc gluconate lozenges shortened the course of a cold.

Zinc nasal sprays are now available and work directly to stop viruses from spreading. If you're already sick, take 13–25 mg of elemental zinc found in zinc gluconate lozenges every two to three hours for five days. According to researchers at Queen's University in Kingston, Ontario, zinc must dissolve in your mouth to work well and is better assimilated when free of sweetening agents like sorbitol or mannitol. Taking zinc for longer than a week may actually weaken immune defenses.

Note: For infants and children, there is some evidence that dietary zinc supplements may reduce the incidence of acute respiratory infections, but this claim is still widely disputed. The best source of zinc for infants and young children is zinc-fortified cereals.

Vitamin E

Vitamin E stimulates the production of natural killer cells that work to seek and destroy germs and cancer cells. Vitamin E also boosts the synthesis of B cells that produce antibodies that target bacteria. Some studies also suggest that vitamin E supplementation may reverse compromised immune function commonly seen in older individuals. It also has significant antioxidant action.

Carotenoid Power

Beta-carotene boosts levels of a variety of infection-fighting immune cells and also works as a powerful antioxidant that scavenges and rounds up dangerous free radicals that can contribute to degenerative diseases and accelerate aging. Beta-carotene also protects cells against cancer by stimulating the action of macrophages that produce tumor necrosis factor (a substance that destroys cancer cells). Beta-carotene supplementation also can increase the production of T lymphocytes and natural killer cells and actually enhances the ability of the natural killer cells to go after and destroy malignant cells. Taking beta-carotene is better than taking vitamin A because beta-carotene converts to vitamin A and is safe even in higher doses, whereas too much vitamin A can be toxic to the body.

Super Selenium

Selenium is a trace element that has remarkable antioxidant properties and also increases natural killer cells and mobilizes cancer-fighting cells. Studies tell us that many Americans are selenium-deficient—a fact that may be related to widespread immune weakness or malfunction.

Fabulous Fatty Acids

There are several studies showing that children taking flaxseed oil every day experienced fewer and less severe respiratory infections and missed fewer days in school. Omega-3 fatty acids found in flaxseed oil and fatty fish (such as salmon, tuna, and mackerel) also increases the activity of phagocytes. These essential fatty acids also protect cells from the toxic waste products of infections. It's best to take vitamin E with an essential fatty acid supplement for maximum benefit.

Get Proactive with Probiotics

Several studies show that the daily consumption of a probiotic lactic acid bacterium (bifidobacterium) optimizes cellular immune responses. Data confirms that taking a probiotic supplement can enhance phagocytosis and natural killer cell activity—an effect that occurs a short time after the consumption of bifidobacteria. Interestingly, this elevated immune activity continued for a time even after supplementation stopped. Good bacteria housed in the colon contributes to disease resistance, and antibiotic therapy can erode good bacteria counts, which need to be replaced with probiotic supplements.

The Maximum Immunity Lifestyle

Providing the body with a diet full of nutrients by eating lots of fresh fruits, vegetables and whole grains is the foundation for good health. In addition, there is no pill that can take the place of a good night's sleep, regular physical activity and lots of laughter, which all work to strengthen the immune system. And don't forget to relieve stress daily. Continuous expo-

Germ Breeding Grounds

Day care centers and nursery schools could also be called germ warfare zones where children can suffer three times as many illnesses as those who stay at home. A study from the *British Medical Journal* suggests that giving a child probiotic lactobacillus (acidophilus) supplementation helps day care kids stay healthy. In addition, because kids are notorious for putting germy objects in their mouths, keeping them supplied with friendly flora fights bacterial fire with (friendly) fire. Several studies show that acidophilus acid bacteria target serious intestinal infections like *E. coli*. And, if your child has been on antibiotics, it's vital to replace the good bacteria that were killed along with the bad. Acidophilus comes in chewable tablets and liquids.

sure to high stress can wear down your resistance to diseases like influenza. Scientists at Carnegie Mellon University in Pittsburgh found that when people with the flu experienced emotional stress, their symptoms got worse. Use regular massage therapy or yoga to diffuse stress and facilitate relaxation. Many of us just don't know how to relax anymore.

Possible Side Effects or Interactions

Glyconutrients have not been found to have significant side effects although polysaccharide-rich herbs like echinacea should not be taken indefinitely. The essential eight sugars are categorized as "foods" but as a rule, if you have any health con-

186 • Miracle Sugars

dition or are taking any medication, you should consult your doctor before taking any supplement. Generally speaking, appropriate supplementation with glyconutrients is considered safe and non-toxic. Anyone with a blood sugar disorder should consult their physician. If you are allergic to yeasts or fungi, you may need to avoid some products. If you experience fast or irregular breathing, skin rash, hives or itching when taking any supplement, call your doctor. You should also consult your doctor before taking any supplement if you have kidney or liver disease, or are pregnant or nursing. At this writing, the safety of these supplements in pregnancy or to infants who are breast-fed has not been established.

Product Availability

First generation sugar sources include a variety of plants, herbs, flowers, gums, fungi and molds. We routinely consumed many of these sugar sources in generations past. Several glyconutrient products can be purchased at health food stores or through product distributors and are considered second generation sugar sources. The essential eight glyconutrients are available in freeze-dried, extracts, loose powder or capsulized forms. They are found in a variety of products from aloe vera supplements to medicinal mushrooms, to sea plants, to herbal combination products designed to boost immune function. Ideally, taking a supplement that provides the best and most complete array of glyconutrients is preferable.

How to Take Glyconutrient-Containing Products

It is generally recommended that the essential eight sugars be taken with food. Powders can be mixed with soft foods or liquids and work better if they are not taken on an empty stomach. The powders can also be placed directly on the tongue. Look for products that are guaranteed, and that offer standardized and stabilized active ingredients. Avoid products that use harsh chemicals like alcohol to extract their compounds. In addition, look for a company telephone number, so you can talk directly to their research and development department if you have any questions or concerns.

References

Adam, E et al. "Pseudomonas aeruginosa II lectin stopshuman cillary beating:therapeutic implications of fucose" American Journal of Respiratory Conditions, Care and Medicine (1997):155(6):2102-2104.

Ahmad, I et al. "Design of liposomes to improve delivery of amphotericin-B in the treatment of aspergillosis" Molc Cellular Biochem (1989 Nov 23-Dec 19):;91(1-2):85-90.

Benoff, S et al. "Induction of the human sperm acrosome reaction with mannose-containing neoglycoprotein ligands" Molecular Human Reproduction (1997 Oct):3(10).

Benton, D. "Case Report: Observed Improvement in Develpmental Dyslexia Accompanied by Supplementation with Glyconutritionals and Phytonutritionals" JANA, Journal of the American Nutraceutical Association (August, 1997): suppl 1, 13-14.

Berger, V et al. "Dietary specific sugars for serum protein enzymatic glycosylation in man" Metabolism (1998 Dec):47(12):1499-503.

Bhavanandan, V "Cancer-associated mucins and mucin-type glycoproteins" Glycobiology (1991 Nov):1(5):493-503.

Bond, A et al. "Distinct oligosaccharide content of rheumatoid arthritis-derived immune complexes" Arthritis and Rheumatism (1995 Jun):38(6):744-9.

Bouhnlk, Y et al "Administration of transgalacto-oligosaccharides increases fecal bifidobacteria and modifies colonic fermentation metabolism in healthy humans" Nutrition (1997):127(3):444-448.

Brandelli, A et al. "Participation of glycosylated residues in the human sperm acrosome reaction: possible role of N-acetylglucosaminidase" Biochem Biophys Acta (1994 Feb 17):1220(3):299-304.

Braaten J et al "Oat beta-glucan reduces blood cholesterol concentration in hypercholesterolemic subjects" European Journal of Clinical Nutrition Jul1994:48(7):465-74.

Brennan, F et al. "TNF alpha—a pivotal role in rheumatoid arthritis?" British Journal of Rheumatolgy (1992):31:293-298.

Brinck, U et al " Detection of Inflammtion and neoplasia associated alterations in human large intestine using plant/invertebrate lectins, glaectin-1 and neoglycoproteins" Acta Anatomica (1998):161: 219-233.

Burmester G et al. "Mononuclear phagocytes and rheumatoid synovitis. Mastermind or workhorse in arthritis?" Arthritis and Rheumatism (1997):40:5-18.

Chandra, R "Nutrition and the immune system: an introduction" American Journal of Clincal Nutrition (1997): 66:460–63S.

Chihara G "Recent progress in immunopharmacology and therapeutic effects of polysaccharides" Developmental Biological Standards 1992;77:191-7.

Cimoch, P et al. "The in vitro immunomodulatory effects of glyconutrients on peripheral blood mononuclear cells of patients with chronic fatigue syndrome" Integrative Physiological and Behavioral Science (1998 Jul-Sep):33(3):280-7.

Clamp, J et al. "Study of the carbohydrate content of mucus glycoproteins from normal and diseased colons" Clinical Science (Colch) (1981 Aug):61(2):229-34.

Crowe, S et al "2-deoxygalactose interferes with an intermediate processing stage of memory", Behavioral and Neural Biology (1994 May):61(3):206-13.

Dabelsteen, E "Cell surface carbohydrates as prognostic markers in human carcinomas" Journal of Pathology (1996 Aug):179(4):358-69.

Davidson M et al "The hypocholesterolemic effects of beta-glucan in oatmeal and oat bran: A dose-controlled study" Journal of the American Medical Association Apr1991:265(14): 1833-9.

de Felippe Junior et al "Infection prevention in patients with severe multiple trauma with the immunomodulator beta 1-3 polyglucose (glucan)" Surgical Gynecology and Obstetrics Oct1993:177(4): 383-8.

Dekaris, D et al. "Multiple changes of immunologic parameters in prisoners of war. Assessments after release from a camp in Manjaca, Bosnia" JAMA Journal of the American Medical Association (1993 Aug 4):270(5):595-9.

Dhurandhar, N "Increased adiposity in animals due to a human virus" Interantional Journal of Obesity and Related Metabolic Disorders (2000 Aug): 24(8):989-96.

Djeraba, A et al. "In vivo macrophage activation in chickens with Acemannan, a complex carbohydrate extracted from Aloe vera" International Journal of Immunopharmacology (2000 May):22(5):365-72.

di Luzio N et al "Comparative evaluation of the tumor inhibitory and antibacterial activity of solubilized and particulate glucan" Recent Results of Cancer Research 1980:75:165-172. "Drug resistance threatens to reverse medical progress" Press Release, WHO World Health Organization/41 (12 June 2000).

Dwek, R et al. "Glycobiology: the function of sugar in the IgG molecule" Journal of Anatomy (1995):187:279-292.

Dykman, Kathryn and Dykman, Roscoe "Effect of Nutritional Supplements on Attention-Deficit Hyperactivity Disorder Integrative Physiological and Behavioral Science" (Jan-March, 1998): 33(1): 49-60.

Dykman, Kathryn and McKinley, Ray "Effects of Glyconutritionals on the Severity of Attention- Deficit Hyperactivity Disorder" Proceedings of the Fisher Institute for Medical Research (November, 1997): 24-25.

Dykman, K et al. "The effects of nutritional supplements on the symptoms of fibromyalgia and chronic fatigue syndrome" Integrative, Physiological and Behavioral Sci (1998 Jan-Mar):33(1):61-71.

Ercan, N et al. "Effects of glucose, galactose, and lactose ingestion on the plasma glucose and insulin response in persons with non-insulin-dependent diabetes mellitus" Metabolism (1993 Dec):42(12):1560-7.

Famularo, G "Infections, atherosclerosis, and coronary heart disease" Annals of the Italian Medical Institute (2000 Apr-Jun):15(2):144-55.

Feizi, T. and Larkin, M "AIDS and glycosylation" Glycobio (Sept 1990): 1(1): 17-23.

Feizi, T. "Significance of Carbohydrate Components of Cell Surfaces, Auto-immunity and Auto-immune diesease" CIBA Foundation, Symposium Series. (United Kingdom: Wiley-Interscience Publications, 1987), 43-57.

Flogel, Lvi et al. "Fucosylation and galactosylation of IgG heavy chains differ between acute and remission phases of juvenile chronic arthritis" Clinical and Chemical Laboratory Medicine (1998):36:99-102.

Forstner, J. "Intestinal mucins in health and disease" Digestion (1978):17(3):234-63.

Fukuda, M "Cell surface carbohydrates: cell-type specific expression. Molecular Glycobiology (Oxford: IRL Press, 1994).

Gardiner, T "Dietary xylose: absorption, distribution, metabolism, excretion (ADME) and biological activity" GlycoScience & Nutrition (2000): 1 (S):1-2.

Gardiner, T "Dietary fucose: absorption, distribution, metabolism, excretion (ADME) and (2000): 1(6): 1-4.

Gardiner, T "Dietary galactose: absorption, distribution, metabolism, excretion (ADME) and (2000): 1(7): 1-4.

Gardiner, T "Dietary N-acetylgalactosamine (GalNAc): absorption, distribution, metabolism, excretion (ADME) and biological activity". GlycoSci & Nutr (2000): 1(8): 1-3.

Gardiner T. Dietary N-acetylneuraminic acid (NANA): absorption, distribution, metabolism, excretion (ADME) and biological activity. GlycoScience & Nutrition 2000; 1(10): 1-3.

Gardiner T. Dietary mannose: absorption, distribution, muetabolism, excretion (ADME) of eight known dietary monosaccharides required for glycoprotein synthesis and cellular recognition processes.

Gardiner, T "Absorption, distribution, metabolism, and excretion (ADME) of eight known dietary monosaccharides required for glycoprotein synthesis and cellular recognition processes: summary" GlycoScience & Nutrition (2000):1(12):1-7.

Gardiner, T "Biological activity of eight known dietary monosaccharides required for glycoprotein synthesis and cellular recognition processes: summary" GlycoScience & Nutrition (2000):1(13):1-4.

Gardiner, T. "Dietary glucose: absorption, distribution, metabolism, excretion (ADME) and biological activity" GlycoScience & Nutrition (2000):1(18):1-4.

Gardiner, T."Glyconutritional implications in fibromyalgia and chronic fatigue syndrome" Glycoscience and Nutrition, (June 3, 2000) 1(21).

Gardiner, T "Gyconutritionals Implications in Failure-to-Thrive Syndrome" Glycoscience and Nutrition,, (2001): 2:1.

Gaspar Y et al "The complex structures of arabinogalactan-proteins and the journey towards understanding function" Plant Molecular Biology 2001 Sep:47(1-2):161-76.

Gauntt, C et al. "Aloe polymannose enhances anti-coxsackievirus antibody titres in mice".phytotherapy Research (2000 Jun):14(4):261-6.

Gauntt, C et al. "Glyconutritionals: Implications for Recovery from Viral Infections" Glycoscience and Nutrition (2001): 2:2.

Ghannoum, M et al. "Protection against Candida albicans gastrointestinal colonization and dissemination by saccharides in experimental animals" Microbios (1991):67(271):95-105.

Gibson, J et al. "Sugar nucleotide concentrations in red blood cells of patients on protein- and lactose-limited diets: effect of galactose supplementation" American Journal of. Clinical Nutrition (1996):63:704-708.

Glaser, R and Kiecolt-Glaser, J "Stress-associated immune modulation: relevance to viral infections and chronic fatigue syndrome" American Journal of Medicine 1998):105(3A):355-425.

Gordon, Garry MD "Heart Disease, America's No. 1 Killer" Explore (1999) 9(4-5).

Grevenstein, J. et al. "Cartilage changes in rats induced by Papain and the influence of treatment with N-acetylglucosamine" Acta P Belgica (1991): 57:2 157-61.

Gupta, J et al "Multiple sclerosis and malabsorption"American Journal of Gastroenterology (1977 Dec):68(6):560-5.

Hakomori, S "Aberrant glycosylation in cancer cell membranes as focused on glycolipids: overview and perspectives" Cancer Research, (1985): 45: 2405-2414.

Hakomori S. "Tumor malignancy defined by aberrant glycosylation and sphingo(glyco)lipid metabolism" Cancer Research (1996 Dec 1):56(23):5309-18.

Hitchen, P et al. "Orientation of sugars bound to the principal C-type carbohydrate-recognition domain of the macrophage mannose receptor" Biochemistry Journal (1998 Aug 1):333(3):601-8 .

"The influence of industrial environmental pollution on the immune system. New ideas of immunorehabilitation " International Conference on Environmental Pollution & Neuroimmunology (1995): 9.

Ironson, G et al "Posttraumatic stress symptoms, intrusive thoughts, loss, and immune function after Hurricane Andrew" Psychosomatic Medicine (1997 Mar-Apr):59(2):128-41.

Jacobs, J and Bovasso, G "Early and chronic stress and their relation to breast cancer" Psychological Medicine (2000 May):30(3):669-78.

Jorgensen, F et al. "Ivlodulation of sialyl Lewis X dependent binding to E-selectin by glycoforms of alpha-i-acid glycoprotein expressed in rheumatoid arthritis" Biomed.Chron (1998):12:343-349.

Josephson L et al "Antiviral activity of a conjugate of adenine-9-beta-D-arabinofuranoside 5'-monophosphate and a 9 kDa fragment of arabinogalactan" Antiviral Therapy 1996 Aug:1(3):147-56.

Kahlon, J et al. "Inhibition of AIDS virus replication by acemannan in vitro" Molecular Biotherapy (1991 Sep):3(3):127-35.

Kai, H et al."Anti-allergic effect of N-acetylneuraminic acid in guinea-pigs" Journal of Pharmaceuticals and Pharmacology (1990 Nov):42(11):773-7.

Kamel, Lvi and Serafi, T "Fucose concentrations in sera from patients with rheumatoid arthritis" Clinical Experimental Rheumatology. (1995): 13:243-246.

Kamel, M et al. "Inhibition of elastase enzyme release from human polymorphonuclear leukocytes by N-acetyl-galactosamine and N-acetyl-glucosamine" Clinical Experimental Rheumatology (1999) 1 9 (9):17-21.

Kelley, D and Daudu, P "Fat intake and immune response" Progressive Food and Nutritional Science (1993)17:41-63.

Klatz, Ronald Adv in Anti-Aging Med, Vol. 1 (Ronald M. Klatz, Editor, 1996), 181-203.

Kobata, Akira "Function and pathology of the sugar chains of human immunoglobulin G. Glycobiology (September 1990), I(1): 5-8.

Kossi, J et al. "Effects of hexose sugars: glucose, fructose, galactose and mannose on wound healing in the rat" Eur Surg Res (1999):31(1):74-82.

Kotler, D et al. "Preservation of short-term energy balance in clinically stable patients with AIDS" American Journal of Clinical Nutrition (1990 Jan):51(1):7-13.

Landin, K et al. "Low blood pressure and blood glucose levels in Alzheimer's disease. Evidence for a hypometabolic disorder" Journal of Internal Medicine (1993 Apr):233(4):357-63.

Lefkowitz, D et al. "Effects of a glyconutrient on macrophage functions" International Journal of Immunopharmacology (2000 Apr):22(4):299-308.

Lefkowitz, Doris "Glyconutritionals: implications for rheumatoid arthritis" Glycoscience and Nutrition (April 15, 2000) 1(16).

Lefkowitz, Doris "Glyconutritionals: Implications in Asthma" Glycoscience and Nutrition, (2000): 1:15.

Lefkowitz, Stanley S. and Lefkowitz,, Doris L. "Glyconutritionals: implications in antimicrobial activity" Glycoscience and Nutrition (2000): 1:22.

Lefkowitz D et al. "Neutrophilic myeloperoxidase-macrophage interactions perpetuate chronic inflammation associated with experimental arthritis" Clinical Inonmomol (1999):91:145-155.

Lhermitte, M et al. "Structures of neutral oligosaccharides isolated from the respiratory mucins of a non-secretor (0, Le a+b-) patient suffering from chronic bronchitis" Glycobiology (June 1991) 1(3): 277-293.

Maihotra, R et al. "Glycosylation changes of IgG associated with rheumatoid arthritis can activate complement via the mannose-binding protein" Nat. Med. (1995):1:237-243.

Mansell P et al et al "Macrophage-mediated destruction of human malignant cells in vivo" Journal of the National Cancer Institute Mar1975:54(3):571-80.

Matsuda, K et al. "Inhibitory effects of sialic acid- or N-acetylglucosamine-specific lectins on histamine release induced by compound 48/80, bradykinin and a polyethylenimine in rat peritoneal mast cells" Japanese Journal of Pharmacology (1994 Jan):64(1):1-8.

Mawle, A et al. "Immune responses associated with chronic fatigue syndrome: a case-control study" Journal of Infectious Diseases (1997):175(1):136-141.

McAnalley, B and Vennum, F "The potential significance of dietary sugars in management of osteoarthritis and rheumatoid arthritis: a review" Proceedings of the Fisher Institute of Medical Research (1997):1:6-10.

McDaniel, Candace, et al. "Effects of Nutraceutical Dietary Intervention in Diabetes Mellitus: A Retrospective Study" Proceedings of the Fisher Institute for Medical Research (November, 1997): 19-23.

Meyer, Walther W. M.D. E-mail: wwm-nutrimed@tds.net

Michaels, E et al. "Effect of D-mannose and D-glucose on Escherichia coli bacteriuria in rats" Urol Res (1983):11(2):97-102.

Mondoa, Emil MD. Sugars That Heal. (Ballantine Books, 2001).

Morikawa K et al et al "Induction of tumoricidal activity of polymorphonuclear leukocytes by a linear beta-1, 3-D-glucan and other immunomodulators in murine cells" Cancer Res. Apr1985:45(4):1496-501.

Moulton, P "Inflammatory joint disease: the role of cytokines, cyclooxygenases and reactive oxygen species" British Journal of Biomedical Science (1996):S3:317-324.

Mullin, B et al. "Myelin basic protein interacts with the myelin-specific ganglioside GM4 Brain Res (1981 Oct 5):222(1):218-21.

Murray, Robert K. Harper's Biochemistry. 24th ed. (Lange, 1996), 648-67.

Olszewski, A et al. "Plasma glucosamine and galactosamine in ischemic heart disease" Atherosclerosis (1990 May):82(1-2):75-83.

Petersen, M et al ."Early manifestations of the carbohydrate-deficient glycoprotein syndrome" Journal of Pediatrics (1993 Jan):122(1):66-70.

Peterson J et al "Glycoproteins of the human milk fat globule in the protection of the breast-fed infant against infections" Biological Neonate 1998:74(2):143-62.

Petruczenko A "Glucan effect on the survival of mice after radiation exposure" Acta Physiol Pol. May1984:35(3):231-6.

Prone Mice" Clinical and Experimental Immunology (Nov. 1996):106: 259-64.

Pugh, N et al. "Characterization of Aloeride, a new high-molecular-weight polysaccharide from Aloe vera with potent immunostimulatory activity" Journal of Agriculture and Food Chemistry (2001 Feb):49(2):1030-4.

Rest, R et al. "Mannose inhibits the human neutrophil oxidative burst" Jour Leukic Biol (1988):43:158-164.

Ringsdorf, W et al"Sucrose, neutrophilic phagocytosis and resistance to disease" Dental Survey (1976):52(12):46.

Robinson R "Effects of dietary arabinogalactan on gastrointestinal and blood parameters in healthy human subjects" Journal of the American College of Nutrition 2001 Aug:20(4):279-85

Ryan, D et al. "GG167 (4-guanidino-2,4-dideoxy-2,3-dehydro-N-acetylneuraminic acid) is a potent inhibitor of influenza virus in ferrets" Antimicrobial Agents and Chemotherapy (1995 Nov):39(11):2583-4.

Rylander R and Lin R "(1—>3)-beta-D-glucan - relationship to indoor air-related symptoms, allergy and asthma" Toxicology Nov 2000:152(1-3):47-52.

Sanchez, A et al. "Role of sugars in human neutrophilic phagocytosis" American Journal of Clinical Nutrition (1973):26:1180.

Sato, R et al. "Substances reactive with mannose-binding protein (lvIBP) in sera of patients with rheumatoid arthritis" Ind Jour Med Sci (1997):43:99-111.

See, D et al. The in vitro immunomodulatory effects of glyconutrients on peripheral blood mononuclear cells of patients with chronic fatigue syndrome" Integrative Physiological and Behavioral Science (1998 Jul-Sep):33(3):280-7.

Smith, B et al. "Analysis of inhibitor binding in influenza virus neuraminidase" Protein Science (2001 Apr):10(4):689-96.

Soltys J et al "Modulation of endotoxin- and enterotoxin-induced cytokine release by in vivo treatment with beta- (1,6)-branched beta- (1,3)-glucan" Infectious Immunology Jan1999;67(1):244-52.

Somasundaram, K and Ganguly, A "Gastric mucosal protection during restraint stress in rats: alteration in gastric adherent mucus and dissolved mucus in gastric secretion" Hepatogastroenterology (1985 Feb): 32(1):24-6.

Stuart, R et al "Upregulation of phagocytosis and candidicidal activity of macrophages exposed to the immunostimulant acemarinan" International Journal of Immunopharmacology (1997):19(2):75-82.

Sullivan, K et al. "Mannose-binding protein genetic polymorphisms in black patents with systemci lupus erythematosus" Arth and Rheumatism (Dec. 1996): 39:12, 2046-51.

Sveinbjornsson B et al "Inhibition of establishment and growth of mouse liver metastases after treatment with interferon gamma and beta-1, 3-D-glucan" Hepatology May1998:27(5):1241-8

Tate, C and Blakely, R "The effect of N-linked glycosylation on activity of the Na(+)- and Cl(-)-dependent serotonin transporter expressed using recombinant baculovirus in insect cells". J.Blol.Clzein. (1994):269(42):26303-26310.

Tazawa K, et al "Anticarcinogenic action of apple pectin on fecal enzyme activities and mucosal or portal prostaglandin E2 levels in experimental rat colon carcinogenesis" Journal of Experimental Clinical Cancer Research 1997 Mar:;16(1):33-8.

Teas J "The dietary intake of Laminarin, a brown seaweed, and breast cancer prevention" Nutrition and Cancer. 1983:4(3):217-22.

Tertov, V et al. "Carbohydrate composition of native and desialylated low density lipoproteins in the plasma of patients with coronary atherosclerosis" Kardiologiia (1992 Sep):32(9-10):57-61.

Trautwein E et al "Effect of different varieties of pectin and guar gum on plasma, hepatic and biliary lipids and cholesterol gallstone formation in hamsters fed on high-cholesterol diets" British Journal of Nutrition 1998 May;79(5):463-71.

Vlietinck, A et al. "Plant-derived leading compounds for chemotherapy of human immunodeficiency virus (HIV) infection" Planta Medica (1998 Mar):64(2):97-109.

Wakui A et al "Randomized study of lentinan on patients with advanced gastric and colorectal cancer" Tohoku Lentinan Study Group Gan To Kagaku Ryoho. Apr1986:13(4 Pt 1):1050-9.

Warczynski, P et al. "Prevention of hepatic metastases by liver lectin blocking with D-galactose in colon cancer patients. A prospectively randomized clinical trial" Anticancer Research (1997 Mar-Apr):17(2B):1223-6.

Warit, S et al."Glycosylation deficiency phenotypes resulting from depletion of GDP-mannose pyrophosphorylase in two yeast species" Molecular Microbiology (2000 Jun):;36(5):1156-66.

Wasser S and Weis A "Therapeutic effects of substances occurring in higher Basidiomycetes mushrooms: a modern perspective" Critical Reviews of Immunology 1999:19(1):65-96.

White, M et al. "Enhanced antiviral and opsonic activity of a human mannose-binding lectin and surfactant protein D chimera" Journal of Immunology (2000 Aug 15):165(4):2108-15.

Wilke,W " Fibromyalgia. Recognizing and addressing the multiple Interrelated factors" Postgraduate Medicine (1996):100(1):153-156.

Wolff, H et al. "Adherence of Escherichia coli to sperm: a mannose mediated phenomenon leading to agglutination of sperm and E. coli" Fertility and Sterility (1993 Jul):60(1):154-8.

Yaqoob, P "Monounsaturated fats and immune function" Proc Nutr Soc (1998):57:511–20.

Yeatman, T et al "Biliary Glycoprotein Is Overexpressed in Human Colon Cancer Cells With High Metastatic Potential" Journal of Gastrointestinal Surgery (1997 May):1(3):292-298.

Index